T0270062

Library of Congress Cataloging-in-Publication Data available upon request.

This book is available in quantity at special discounts for your group or organization. For further information, contact:

Triumph Books LLC
814 North Franklin Street
Chicago, Illinois 60610
(312) 337-0747
www.triumphbooks.com

Printed in U.S.A.

ISBN: 978-1-63727-649-5
Design by Patricia Frey

All images courtesy of Christi Williford, Elemental Studio Design

To my amazing wife, Christine.
Thank you for pushing me to write this book
and for your unwavering support. There is no
one else with whom I'd rather do burpees!

Contents

Introduction vii

1. Owning Your Fitness Journey 1

2. Adaptation Cycle 23

3. Are You Ready to Train? 41

4. Strength Training 69

5. Fitness Check-up 81

6. Your Fit Score 103

7. Lifestyle and Nutrition 113

8. Creating Your Fitness Plan 151

9. Workout Design Overview 179

Appendix

   A. Single-Sided Balance and Stability Exercises 193

   B. Additional Assessments and Fixes 197

   C. Hypermobility, Isometric Exercises, Eccentric
      Training, and Instability 205

   D. Mobility for Sitting Too Much 211

   E. Carb Cycling and Nutrition Resources 213

   F. Higher-Level Fitness Tests 219

   G. Specific Exercises to Improve Your Fit Score 223

   H. Additional (Fun!) Challenges 229

Citations 231

Acknowledgments 239

Introduction

Most of us have a movement practice, whether it's running, Pilates, group fitness, or a mix of things. And for years that might have been enough to keep us at our desired level of health and fitness. But as we age, what worked in our 20s and 30s no longer has the same effect. Between the ages of 40 and 59, most of us will gain more body fat than at any other point in our lives.[1] When we reach 40 years old, production of sex hormones begins to decrease by up to 3 percent per year, so even if we are active and show up to the gym, we will face changing hormone levels that will affect our body composition, mood, energy, and overall health.[2] When we reach middle age, we can no longer just check the box when it comes to fitness and wellness. We need a new set of tools that will support impactful and sustainable change.

The truth is, as we get older we need different things from our fitness practice. And in order to understand those needs, we need to understand the art and science behind exercise. It's not as easy as simply changing things up when something stops working. Instead, the answer lies in understanding what you, individually, need in order to continue to see change.

My fitness career has been spent with one foot in professional sports—first as a professional soccer player and later as the head of performance for several Olympic and professional athletes and the head strength and conditioning coach for Minnesota United Football Club—and the other foot in the group fitness and personal training industry. My wife, Christine, and I have owned and operated FIT Studio, a boutique gym in Minneapolis, for 22 years. I have also worked on the corporate side of the fitness industry with Anytime Fitness as part of their operations team, where I helped support growth in personal training and group fitness. My passion is to help support a new fitness paradigm in gyms, clinics, and communities, and give individuals the information they need to chase their own fitness now and into the future.

Many people who show up at our studio have tried everything—they've checked all the boxes. They've tried what worked for their friend or neighbor or celebrity spokesperson, but it didn't work for them. They trained with the guy who promised weightlifting or HIIT or yoga was *the* answer. They embraced the latest fad diet and exercise craze. They wanted to lose 10 lbs or get faster or set a new personal record or be leaner, but they're stuck.

They're stuck because no one taught them how to take a shot at solving their own health and fitness problems. No one explained how to set up a training week based on their specific body type, age, sex, goals, emotions, injuries, and fitness level. (Yes, all of these things come into play.) My first job is to help them understand that there isn't one practice or one plan that works for everyone. We are all different, so we need different things, different approaches.

My job is to teach them how to curate their own fitness experience, how to put the disparate pieces together.

Take Peter, who showed up at our studio about ten years ago. Peter referred to himself as "the most in-shape fat guy" you'd ever meet. At the time, Peter was in his mid-40s and had a fitness routine that looked solid on paper. On Mondays he did a fast 3-mile run. Tuesdays he took a Pilates class, which he called his strength day. Wednesday was a spin workout at a local fitness studio. Thursday was a longer, slow run. Friday was his boot camp class at a different local studio. Saturday and Sunday were off or he went on a long run one of the days. Peter loved his weekly routine and stuck to it week in and week out. But when he was in his early 40s he began to notice that his weight and body fat were going up. By the time he got to me, he was 20 lbs heavier than he had been five years earlier. He could still hit it pretty hard in the gym and on a run, but something wasn't working. Peter's body had not only adapted to what he was doing, meaning it was no longer changing with the exercise he was doing, but he seemed to be going backward with his health. Peter assumed that, even as he aged, if he kept up with his routine, he'd stay fit.

Peter was missing some key elements in his weekly routine. Helping Peter understand where the holes were, how to begin the process of filling those holes, and giving him the ability to make adjustments as he went along, was what allowed Peter to lose his 20 lbs and then another 10 lbs and get into the best shape of his life. A decade later, Peter is still chasing fitness, still highly engaged in his practice, and constantly making the adjustments he now knows how to make to continue to grow.

We all get stuck sometimes—emotionally and physically—in life and in our fitness. I am no exception. For most of my life, what I did for fitness worked. When I played professional soccer, I trained daily and was at peak fitness. Later, I learned to love being in a gym, running, biking, lifting weights, and being active outdoors. But then, in early 2023, at the age of 49, I was diagnosed with cancer.

The surgery and treatment stopped me in my tracks. Over three months, I went from active, strong, and energized to sedentary, tired, and frail. My treatment plan included taking a drug that blocks the hormones that feed my specific kind of cancer. This forced me into male menopause. It was as if I had aged 20 years overnight. I lost 20 lbs of muscle, developed a belly, and lost my desire to train. I also experienced night sweats, anxiety, and depression. All I wanted to do was sleep and eat processed carbs. I was more than stuck; I was miserable.

I tried returning to my old training plan of five days a week, which included heavy lifting and aggressive cardio, but I no longer had the energy for hour-long strength sessions that combined upper body, lower body, and a short HIIT session. The old way was getting me nowhere. I needed to simplify my plan.

I had all the tools I needed to get unstuck. After all, I had helped thousands of clients figure out how to do just that. But I was still reeling from my diagnosis and I was worried. I knew that strength training was the only way to increase my hormone production energy levels and reverse the effects of menopause, but what if the change in hormone levels due to strength training actually increased my risk of cancer recurrence?

I talked to my oncologist and learned that high intensity training and weightlifting can regulate insulin and estrogen levels, which is good in preventing certain cancers, including mine. I also learned that the increase in lean muscle associated with an increase in testosterone and human growth hormone actually reduces the risk of most cancers because it boosts the immune system, increases the metabolism, and reduces fat. Clearly, these benefits far outweighed the alternative of either doing nothing or relying on medication alone.

So I picked two days a week and focused on building my way back to doing heavier strength training. I was weak initially, but I'd created a plan that would progress slowly. The short-term response in hormones woke me up, made me feel more alert, and helped with my anxiety and depression. After two weeks, the night sweats were gone, my mood stabilized, and I stopped losing muscle. I once again loved training and looked forward to my workouts. I was, thankfully, unstuck.

My goal as a performance coach, personal trainer, and teacher has always been to help my athletes understand the things they need to know in order to make themselves better and get themself unstuck. I want them to be critical thinkers about their own fitness. I have helped hundreds of professional athletes competing at the highest level understand how to eat, how to sleep, how to train, and how to recover year after year in order to be at their best. And I use the same principles of science to help my clients in the studio be in the best shape of their lives.

It is every person's right to be educated about how to use exercise not just to be healthy, but to chase fitness as far as they want. Chasing fitness applies to everyone and simply means that you are identifying what is important to you, looking ahead to what's next for your health and fitness, and following a fitness and wellness progression that makes the most sense for you in this specific moment. It will be different for everyone, but with the right tools and an understanding of how to apply those tools, you can reach your wellness goals.

The New Fit will help you close the gap that exists between where the science of sport lives and where group fitness, personal training, and general fitness lives, and put all the pieces together in order to create a lifelong practice that constantly changes and evolves as *you* evolve. Don't worry—you won't need expensive new equipment or the latest gadgets; you will be able to utilize your resources at home, in your gym, and online. And I won't ask you to stop getting on your Peloton or working with your trainer. I will simply help you curate your experience by giving you the knowledge you need to add the right things to your fitness practice in order to make impactful changes.

This book will help you become a critical thinker in your own fitness journey and help you reframe the way you look at exercise. You will learn how to take vital fitness assessments so you know where you fit in the larger picture of fitness and you will learn how to progress. I will provide a clear day-to-day path forward that explains and tailors training, movement, and nutrition. You will come to understand your fitness and nutritional needs, not based on what worked for someone else, but what will work for you based on your background, sex, age, genetics, and interests. And I'll teach you how to identify if it's working or not and how to tweak it until you are at a place where you are seeing results and moving forward.

Welcome! I hope you learn, enjoy, and connect with the resources in this book in a way that helps you embark on an impactful wellness journey that fits your needs now and into the future.

CHAPTER 1

Owning Your Fitness Journey

My wife, Christine, was an excellent high jumper in high school, able to jump six feet, which earned her an NCAA Division I scholarship to Illinois State University. In high school, Christine also ran and trained for the 400-meter sprint. A big part of Christine's high-jump technique was her ability to generate speed as she approached the bar, so a sprinting practice kept her fit and helped her speed, both of which made her a better high jumper. But when she got to ISU, which, in the mid-90s, was a big NCAA program with little individualized training, her coach focused solely on jumping. He didn't want his jumpers to do any running. For some of the jumpers, doing no speed work or any conditioning worked well. Their bodies responded nicely, and that's what they needed to thrive. For Christine, this approach didn't work. She needed speed work and conditioning to stay at her peak. She didn't improve without it and struggled to jump her previous heights.

Different athletes need different ways to train so that they thrive. What worked for one athlete might not work for another. Some people can't run, but they can bike. Some people need more strength-driven workouts, while others need more cardio. This is why group fitness and training apps, where everyone does the same intervals for the same amount of time with the same intensity cues, don't work for everyone.

If you want to thrive and eventually see change, even as you age, you must consider age and sex, hormones, tolerance for intensity, time for recovery, and purpose of training. You'll need to consider why you like what you like in your movement practice and why you fear or dread the things you avoid or are unwilling to try. Fitness is emotional. It can be scary to work out. It can be intimidating to walk into a gym. It can be frustrating dealing with injuries. But fitness is also a great place to get to know yourself and understand who you are, what drives you and what keeps you connected. Understanding your limits—the point at which you fail—is part of the process, and yes, that can be scary, but it's also exciting.

Are you willing to take a close look at who you are—to look under the hood, so to speak—in order to embrace your fitness journey in a meaningful way? When you actively participate in your fitness and the decision-making process for yourself and your wellness, you will be able to solve the problems keeping you stuck and get to know yourself better in the process. Three key factors play a part for those who thrive in their fitness: **awareness, connection, and progression.**

Awareness

Sometimes it takes something big to make us stop and take an in-depth look at what we are doing and why we are doing it. Maybe it's a pre-diabetes diagnosis, high cholesterol levels, weight gain, menopause, or a chronic condition that forces us to reassess. When this happens, we go from being bystanders to critical thinkers about our health and wellness, gathering as much information as possible. The big question is why do most of us need these wake-up calls in order to be aware and engaged in our health practices?

When we're comfortable in our fitness routines, environments, and communities, it's easy to just keep showing up and doing the same thing even if we're not progressing or even maintaining our fitness levels. Comfort and community are important and they are powerful! But as aging fitness consumers, we have to be more aware, more engaged, and more knowledgeable so that we can continue to be fit and active as we grow older.

Being around professional athletes has given me insight into the instinct to welcome discomfort as part of the growth process. One of the most commonly identifiable traits of the best teammates and athletes is that they have learned to look forward to challenges and discomfort because they know it makes them better and brings out the best in them. A good competitor thrives in discomfort and adversity because they want to take on the challenge. The greater the challenge, the greater the reward.

It's the same with fitness. It requires grit, determination, and hard work to make fitness work. Notice I said nothing about athleticism or ability. You don't need to be able to run an eight-minute mile or do 25 burpees in a minute. That's great if you can, but it's not really about those results; it's about your willingness to deal with adversity and challenge. Not everyone steps into their fitness journey with the skill of hard work, but it is something that you'll learn in the following chapters.

It's helpful to know what type of person you are when it comes to training. There are basically two types of people: the overtraining type and the undertraining type. The people who overtrain tend to get stuck in a pattern that is never high-reaching enough to force change. These people usually function at a pretty high level, but they are stuck. I know it sounds contradictory that the overtraining type never reaches high enough, but they usually overwork themselves so they are never fully rested and ready to train, thus they are not able to reach high enough intensity in their exercise. This group doesn't feel they need rest because they never actually get the intensity intended and they have forgotten what it feels like to be rested and ready, so their intensity scale is off. This cycle leads them into the black hole of training, and nothing ever changes.

Often, the people in this category are addicted to doing some form of exercise almost every day. Many are former athletes who grew up in athletic environments where the message was "more is always better." This category also includes people who were once sedentary and unfit, then had a fitness awakening that helped them get out of that slump, but they never were taught that eventually what they were doing would have to change, so they just keep driving deeper and deeper into their commitment. And the thought of recovering in order to reach higher is too scary because they don't want to risk taking a day off because they fear they will go back to their old sedentary ways.

Linda was the overtraining type. She wanted to train hard every day. She had been an athlete in college and was used to associating the feeling of hard training with accomplishment and results. She could train hard almost every day in her twenties and thirties, but when she got into her mid-late forties, her body started to change, she was constantly tired, and she was losing her desire to work out. She was no longer getting stronger, faster, and leaner. She went from loving the challenge of running faster and lifting heavier weights to dreading going to the gym or heading out for a run. Her solution was to commit more, dig harder, and push through. But what Linda really needed was an overhaul in her program that included taking days off or training less intensely on certain days.

Previously, Linda combined strength training with cardio, thinking it made her workouts more challenging, but instead she was diluting both her strength and cardio training. She did deadlifts, then ran two minutes, came back and did more deadlifts, and would repeat this cycle. But by doing this, she was stealing from her own intensity; her two-minute runs were not very fast because she was tired from the deadlifts and the deadlifts weren't strong because she was tired from the running.

By separating the two types of exercise, she could be more effective in each. She quickly got stronger and faster because each became more potent. There is nothing wrong with mixing elements like deadlifting and running in the same workout. But as we age we also must consider the importance of taking the time to work on specific elements in order to see progress. Combining practices might be fun, but sometimes we need to pull those elements apart and just focus on one in order to see improvement. It's no different than building a skill in sport. You don't always show up to practice and play a scrimmage. Sometimes you work on basic skills or skill development in order to get better overall.

After Linda separated her strength and cardio training, she was no longer in the gym for 90 minutes each day; instead, she was in the gym for 45–60 minutes each weekday and she took Saturday and Sunday off. If she wanted to do something active over the weekend, the rule was that it couldn't have anything to do with training. It had to be recreational fun, like taking a bike ride, playing a sport with friends, or trying something new. With her new plan in place, Linda once again looked forward to getting into the gym, she was getting stronger and leaner, and she had more energy.

LINDA	
Monday	STRENGTH
Tuesday	EASY LONG CARDIO
Wednesday	STRENGTH
Thursday	SPRINTS
Friday	WALK
Saturday	SLEEP IN / RECOVERY
Sunday	REST OR PLAY

The undertraining type differs from the overtraining type, but the outcome is similar; both have very little change in performance or body composition. The driving factor behind the pattern, however, is different. The undertraining type is usually unaware of their ability and/or they have a lower tolerance for intensity. They have not yet tested the boundaries of their capacity regarding exercise intensity. Not knowing how high they can actually reach, they will never get to the high peaks of intensity where they teeter on failure and experience true discomfort, so they never need recovery time. They, too, go through the motions, but for different reasons than the overtraining type.

Often, people in this category don't have a background to pull from that allows them to connect to intensity. Maybe they didn't play sports or they aren't used to going outside their comfort zone. Maybe they never dealt with discomfort and didn't recognize the feeling, or conversely, maybe they experienced a great deal of discomfort—physical or emotional—in their lives and they are extremely averse to putting themselves back in that physical and emotional state. Studies have shown that hospitalized children report needle procedures as one of their most feared and painful experiences. Needle-related fear may result in increased avoidance behavior and attempts to eliminate any possible exposure to needles.[3] The same goes for adults who have a fear of discomfort— they will avoid it whenever possible.

Whereas the overtraining types are limited by lack of rest and recovery time, undertraining types are limited by the lack of intensity that they pull into their fitness routine. Do not confuse this with a lack of athleticism. It's easy to think that the overtraining type is athletic and the undertraining type is unathletic. That's not accurate. Regardless of athleticism, genetics, and experience, you will be successful in chasing fitness if you can learn to do hard things. Not hard things in the gym, not great-feats-of-athleticism hard things, just the ability to push through. If you have drive and determination to get through hard things, it makes this journey easier.

Types of Trainers

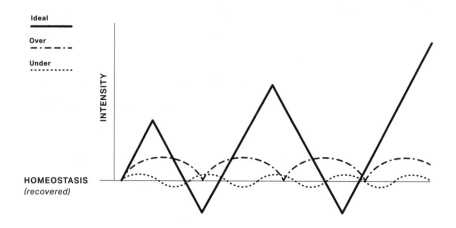

Some of us don't like discomfort, but discomfort is where we grow, so part of this journey is about learning to deal with discomfort. For some that's easier than others, and there is a plan to help everyone not only understand where they fall on this scale, but how to get better at being able to do hard things. You can see how important understanding your emotional connection to discomfort is as you look at training. Some of you want to jump into intensity and testing the boundaries, but others might need a more careful approach that allows for more reflection, practice, and patience.

I've found the best way to help yourself as an undertraining type is to build out a simple program that measures progression over a short amount of time. This allows you to start from a comfortable place but with a plan that will lead you toward the right dose of intensity. If you used 10 lbs this week, use 12 lbs next week, and so on. I'll be more specific later in the book, but know that if you identify as an undertraining type, having a progressive plan is critical. The plan allows you to see what's coming, which can remove some of the apprehension and fear. Eventually your training will become challenging, but the slow ramp up is helpful. The key, again, is to understand that you'll have to risk failure to understand what you are really capable of. Failure doesn't happen on Day 1. Over time you'll edge closer to it, and by the time you get there, you'll be ready for it. Failure is where learning and growth takes place, it goes from being scary to providing clarity and progression. Building slowly toward failure in a planned systematic way can feel safer.

Take Amy, for example. Amy wasn't accustomed to failure as part of her fitness practice. She showed up, trained, and went home without ever getting out of breath or really pushing toward the edge of her capabilities. She was consistent and understood nutrition, but she just couldn't find a way forward to see change. Her plan consisted of taking different fitness classes she liked. If she couldn't do that, she would do a YouTube dance video at home. Amy was uncertain about doing hard things in the gym because it wasn't familiar to her, she was afraid of how it felt to go to the edge, to get out of breath and feel her heart pound.

I knew that in order for Amy to see change and progress, she would have to be willing to go through hard things physically, and she would have to learn to embrace those challenges in order for it to be a sustainable part of her practice. Understanding the science behind intensity and failure helped, but Amy was still not ready to jump in. She needed a plan to slowly ease her way into discomfort so that she could learn to trust herself in situations that felt uncomfortable. In the end, it was Amy's awareness of herself and her response to the physical feeling of intensity that allowed her to get past her fear. We started by getting her out of breath for just a few seconds. Those opportunities gave her confidence that she would be okay. Slowly, 10 seconds of being out of breath turned into one minute and then two minutes. Eventually, Amy got to the point that being out of breath was something she no longer feared, and instead looked forward to, and she was able to do things that she'd never done before. She could do interval runs, where she would run fast for a few minutes, get out of breath, then rest and go again. She embraced running, strength training, and doing hard things, and as a result, she lost over 20 lbs. More importantly, her training went from something she just showed up for, to an experience with which she was fully engaged.

Something that helps people realize what the right dose of intensity is for them is by learning about fitness standards for others their age who are strong, healthy, and fit. Again, I'm not talking about the people who live and breathe fitness, who break records and dedicate everything to being fit. I'm talking about people who have figured out how to see their fitness journey differently and, in turn, have changed. In particular, I have found that it helps the undertraining type see the gap between what they are doing and what can be done by other people who are in their shoes but are now fit. We will discuss this in detail in Chapters 5 and 6, which will provide you with fitness markers.

Connection

Connection is an absolutely necessary step in establishing a sustainable practice. Being connected to your movement practice means that you have found something you love doing, something you're passionate about, something at which you want to improve. It's not enough to just like it. That won't make you want to improve, dig in, and get excited about showing up daily. Certainly, you have something in your life that you are connected to, something you think about when you're not doing it, something at which you desire to be better. My mom, who is from Mexico and is Jewish, loves cooking. As a kid, I spent hours mixing, stirring, and tasting everything from traditional homemade taquitos to homemade matzah ball soup. Those memories bring me joy, and though I didn't realize it then, those experiences as a kid in my mom's kitchen gave me a foundation for my love of cooking.

It wasn't until I had kids of my own that it all came together. I would sit my kids on the counter and they would help me cook and bake. Often, my mom would be on speaker phone guiding us through a special family recipe. I didn't always get it right. The food was sometimes overcooked or not seasoned correctly, but it didn't matter. Because it wasn't really about the food; it was the love, the passion, and the connection that went into making each meal. Now, my kitchen is stocked with cookbooks, different types of pots and pans, and specialty cooking tools. I love to watch cooking shows to learn new recipes and techniques. As a family, we are always trying new recipes and we invent quite a few of our own. Not everything always comes out the way we want it, but I've realized that cooking for us is much less about the result and more about the connection and the experience.

This kind of connection is what everyone must find in their movement practice. It doesn't have to be in a gym or on a bike, but take the basic elements you hear me describing in my connection to cooking and think about your movement practice to see if you are connected, passionate, always wanting to improve, looking forward to participating, more driven by the experience than the results. That connection is crucial in having a sustainable and effective movement practice.

If you don't have a practice that you are connected to, try the following:

1. Be open to trying new things. Experiment and pay attention to how you feel before, during, and after exercise. It's not always a linear path to find a movement practice to which you are connected. It takes time.

2. Be honest with yourself. It can be easy to get caught up in the latest fitness fad or what worked for someone else. Find your own path forward. Think about sustainability. Is this something you can see yourself doing over time?

3. Look to the past. If you felt connected to a movement or exercise in the past, you will likely be able to connect to it again. I am connected to cooking because I grew up in a home where I helped my mom cook as a child and loved it. What did you do in the past for movement, sport, or exercise that you loved? That is your starting point. Maybe it's being outside in nature, maybe it's a sport you used to play, maybe you remember the feeling you had bonding with

teammates, or the connection you felt with a parent when you kicked a ball in the backyard.

4. It's about you. Don't worry about what anyone else says or thinks. Just find a connection. You'll feel it in your body.

A decade ago, Stacy arrived in the studio. Stacy was a 48-year-old mom and had tried everything—every diet and every workout program. She knew more about nutrition and fitness than most trainers. She'd tried every detox, paleo, and vegan diet you could think of, but she couldn't get the results she wanted. She had tried Pure Barre training, Pilates, yoga, and CrossFit, but nothing ever stuck. She just couldn't seem to authentically connect to what she tried.

Stacy signed up for group fitness at our gym and she jumped in enthusiastically, swinging a kettlebell, sprinting, and using a barbell. But after about two weeks, she stopped showing up. It wasn't until we sat down to talk about what was going on that she recognized a pattern: she would jump all in but then realize she just wasn't connected and suddenly stop. There was no joy, passion, love, or excitement for her in these movement practices. She only did them because she thought they might help her lose weight and be fitter.

She was externally motivated and thought that each "next thing"—next diet, next fitness fad—would be the answer. This is the opposite of being internally motivated to change. I asked her to share with me the parts of her day that involved movement that she liked and to describe the exercise she'd done in the past that she liked. She loved walking her dog and going on bike rides; she felt connected to these practices. I helped Stacy understand the importance of enjoying and looking forward to what you do daily for your movement practice.

It wasn't an easy transition for Stacy; she still wanted to lose weight by doing what she saw people around her doing: going to the gym, signing up for endurance races, and adopting crazy diets. She had to work at slowing down and understanding that first she had to enjoy what she was doing. I worked with Stacy to help her identify her goals and also understand her needs for her body type, age, and experience.

With that knowledge, she created a practice anchored in the things she loved. And once Stacy was able to connect to and enjoy her movement practice, it didn't take long for her to desire progression. Her walks with her dog turned into runs with her dog. Her bike rides progressed to mountain biking for sport and competition. It happened naturally, as it does for anyone with a passion for something. Her desire to become a better, stronger, more competitive mountain biker brought her back to the gym for the right reasons. She began to feel better emotionally—about herself and beyond, which was so gratifying. And eventually, she did lose the desired weight, but that was a by-product of her connection with mountain biking, not the focus of her training. Stacy was able to find what she connected with and build a progressive, sustainable plan around what she loved.

Dr. Rick Aberman, the former sports psychologist for the Minnesota Twins, explains how using connection and passion for sport can help professional teams select the right athletes to recruit and sign. He explains there often can be more value in choosing the athlete who is connected, passionate, and wants to improve in their sport rather than the athlete who is just big and strong but might not be as driven to be better. The long-term outcomes are usually better when you put together a group of athletes who love what they're doing and want to improve instead of just wanting to win. The same applies to you as you look at your fitness practice. Find what you are passionate about, what you want to improve at, and what makes you feel good. This creates the foundation for an impactful long-term fitness practice.

Progression

Over all the years I've worked with professional athletes, not once has one of them shown up to practice and said, "I have arrived. I'm the best in the world, so I don't need to practice anymore." Not even Kristina Koznick, who, when I worked with her, was the best female slalom skier in the world, with six World Cup wins and three Olympic appearances. She was the best, and still she wanted to get better. She was always challenging herself, always thinking of what was next and what she needed to improve on.

Kristina had the desire to progress because she loved alpine ski racing; she was connected with what she did. She loved the competition, the challenge, and working to get better. Winning was a by-product of all this. Kristina's desire to always be better was something about which she was passionate. It wasn't stressful; it was challenging and engaging. She looked forward to each day of training and competition because she wanted to see what she could do, what she was capable of, how she was improving, and what new things she would learn. Kristina's fitness progression was a key element in continuing to develop as a skier even later in her career. I remember getting off the slopes with her at training camp at Mammoth Mountain in California. Everyone was done for the day and had packed up and headed inside. Kristina wanted to run a dryland session right there in the parking lot, so I got out medicine balls, plyo boxes, and kettlebells and we did it. At 30 years old, in her final Olympic appearance in Italy, she was still progressing.

We all have to look at our movement practice in the same way. If you aren't chasing fitness and wellness, if there is no progression in your practice, then you will, eventually, become stuck. Maybe you've been doing the same thing week after week, month after month, and year after year, and it's worked for you. That's great! But as you age, the same thing that worked once will no longer work. At some point, your body will adapt, and you might start to get bored or not see results anymore. You will likely lose strength, gain body fat, and see a decrease in overall fitness. You might even lose the desire to train.

Once you find something you are connected to, you need a progression that goes along with that practice. Progression does three main things for all of us in our movement practice. One, it provides a clear path forward. That clarity makes it easy to know what direction you are heading and what results might be expected at each marker. For example, if I run a 10-minute mile and my goal is to run an eight-minute mile, my plan to progress has specific markers. First I have to get to a 9:30-minute mile, then a nine-minute mile, and so on. This is different from simply showing up each day to work out. This gets rid of any ambiguity, which helps in remaining focused.

Two, it provides motivation. Always having something in front of you to chase can be motivating if you're chasing it for the right reasons. For Kristina, her internal motivation drove her to want to be better. She was well-grounded and connected to her progression and wanted to be the best for herself. When things didn't go her way, or she didn't win, she was okay because she wasn't chasing the win. She was chasing progression and improvement. This is where many of us in fitness get stuck. We are chasing a result, which makes it hard because we are connected to the result, which is outside our control. When our passion and connection are in our practice, and we truly love what we are doing for exercise, it's easy to be present and see what challenge is in front of us. The progression is just about getting better at what you do. The by-product is winning the race or losing the 10 lbs.

This is not the way society portrays fitness. If you search "fitness" on Instagram, you will find images of six packs and minimally clothed people with lean bodies. If this is what you are chasing, it's not going to last. Find what you want internally, what is healthy, what is meaningful to you on a personal level, and your fitness will be much easier to connect with, and thus, easier to progress and sustain.

Three, progression provides efficacy. As we watch ourselves improve, we know that we are choosing the right things to do for fitness. If we don't see improvement, we must change the path. It's like running an experiment on yourself. It can be broken down into five simple steps, all of which I will walk you through later in the book: 1) have a measurable goal; 2) come up with a plan; 3) start running your experiment; 4) see if it's working; and 5) make adjustments based on what you are learning and apply the science.

When I met David in his early forties, he was connected to the type of exercise he was doing and he was constantly getting better. He was healthy and felt great. But then David's job became more demanding, and he got stuck in his fitness regimen. He still ran or got on his Peloton most days of the week and he was connected to those movement practices. He was a clean eater and consumed minimal alcohol. On paper, everything looked decent, but David had been doing the same thing for about five years, and he was gaining body fat and losing muscle. His cholesterol was up, and his blood pressure was rising, as well.

When David came to see me in his early fifties, he couldn't see a clear path forward. He needed a fitness plan that would allow him to progress. A plan based on progression ensures that we are doing the right things in the right order at the right intensities. Running and Peloton were still part of his plan—David loved both of those practices—but we changed his Monday workout to strength training. Sunday was David's off day, and at his age, he needed more lean muscle to increase his metabolism and lower his body fat, so I wanted him to go into the strength session after a day of rest. Previously, strength training was an afterthought for David; he left it until the end of the week when he was already tired. That meant the strength work wasn't potent enough to support the change he was seeking.

A big part of progression is the increase in intensity over specific time intervals. Intensity comes in many forms: speed, load, and time. For David, the specific type of intensity he needed as a 53-year-old male was the load. He needed the stimulus from lifting heavy loads to increase hormone production and, therefore, increase metabolism and lean muscle and decrease body fat. For the first few weeks, we worked on making sure David could squat appropriately, pain-free and with good mechanics. Then we added speed, making sure he could stay connected and strong in the movement. Finally, he added load, which he increased each week. David ended up enjoying the strength training sessions so much that he replaced one of his running days with strength training. He continued to progress over the next year and eventually lost 15 lbs, dropped 7 percent of his body fat, and returned his cholesterol and blood pressure to healthy levels. But what was most important to David was that he had connected to a new way of thinking about fitness and now he had the knowledge to continue to progress on his own.

The science of sport helps change outcomes. Athletes get stronger and faster by following the science. But sustainable fitness is more than just science; it's emotion, connection, and passion. When you find the right combination of science and connection you will see change. When we are open to learning, to looking at our fitness in a different way, we expand our knowledge and become more aware of what might work for us on an individual level. This is how we start owning our fitness and building the skills to make informed decisions for ourselves.

CHAPTER 2
Adaptation Cycle

Whether you have a strict fitness plan you follow each day or you move based on whatever the day brings, keep moving. You are healthier for it, and moving puts you in the top 17 percent of the U.S. population if you are over 40.[4] But as I mentioned earlier, as we age, most of us gain weight and lose muscle. So if you keep doing the same thing you are doing now for fitness, it will eventually stop working. You'll need to change the way you are doing your fitness to surpass the rate at which your body is deteriorating. That's where the adaptation theory, which is the idea of organizing and individualizing our fitness in order to see positive changes, comes in.

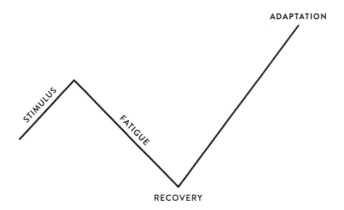

Adaptation is when the body adapts to a stimulus, like exercise. How you adapt to a stimulus depends on many factors, including your fitness starting point. For example, if you were sedentary and overweight and you started training for a 5K race by running for the first time in a long time (running being the stimulus), you might see weight loss occur (weight loss being the adaptation). If you already have a movement practice but feel stuck and are not seeing your body adapt anymore, you will need a stronger or different stimulus. You may need to add intensity, load, speed, and variation, or you may need to add more recovery if you are overtraining. Most likely, it's a combination of all of these. In order to understand how to fix what's keeping you stuck, you need to understand the adaptation cycle.

Adaptation takes place in four phases—stimulus, fatigue, recovery, and adaptation—and these phases make up the adaptation cycle. The adaptation cycle allows us to apply true science to fitness and find efficacy in any training program. If what you are doing doesn't follow the four phases of adaptation, it might be good, but it's not as effective as it could be. Using the four phases of adaptation is the foundation of impactful, meaningful training with an individualized purpose and goal. These four phases of adaptation are at the core of how we shift the way we look at fitness. Once you understand what goes into forcing the body to change, you will see that all training must have a purpose with specific peaks in intensity and dips for recovery. We all adapt to different stimuli in different ways and, along with that, we all need different amounts of recovery.

Keep in mind that each step of adaptation is dependent on the step before it. No phase in the cycle can be isolated; each phase, in order, is necessary to see change. You may need to be open to adding to, subtracting from, or changing what you currently do to see change. Don't worry, you don't have to completely throw out what you're doing now, but my hope is that by understanding how adaptation works, you'll be able to tweak or reinvent a movement practice so that you can move forward and understand how to get your body to adapt as you age.

As we go through these four phases of the adaptation cycle, I will reiterate the fact that fitness is emotional. We all bring outside patterns to fitness, and because fitness is stressful not only physically but emotionally, our patterns tend to be exaggerated with fitness. For example, I am very non-committal, ask any of my friends. If you invite me to go on a walk, or hang out, or go to watch a soccer game, it's difficult for me to commit. I'm afraid if I do, I'll miss out on something else. I've had the same issue with my fitness. I know that just waking up each day and coming up with whatever workout I feel like doing doesn't work for me, but in the past I had the tendency to do that because I was afraid if I followed a pre-designed program, I'd miss out on something that might help me more with my fitness. But I've realized that if I don't track my training, if I don't have a plan, if I just do whatever, I usually end up getting injured, overdoing it, and burning out after a few weeks. When I plan my fitness, I might not always get to do what I feel like I should or want to do, but I do what I *need* to do and the results are so much better. So just be aware of what patterns you are bringing to your fitness; this will help you address any blind spots you have.

Now let's dive into the phases of the adaptation cycle.

Phase 1: The Stimulus

The stimulus is what you do for exercise. The type of exercise we do as we age is a key factor in fat loss, metabolism, and overall wellness. Balance in your fitness practice is also important. Moderate, longer aerobic exercise has a catabolic effect on your body, meaning going for a run or doing a cardio Peloton class sends a message to the body to break down the body's protein stores, which means eating muscle. But cardiovascular endurance training also uses fat as fuel, and thus supports lower blood pressure, better cholesterol levels, and stronger heart and lungs. In contrast, strength training has an anabolic effect, meaning doing the right type of strength training can increase hormone production, which needs to be a strong consideration as you age.

Hormones significantly influence how our bodies adapt. Both men and women have testosterone and estrogen, along with many other hormones that are key in maintaining lean muscle, healthy metabolism, strong bones, good energy levels, and so many other things that allow us to stay strong, healthy, and age well. Those hormones are affected differently by the different exercises we do. So, as we look at stimulus, especially in those of us over 40, which is when our hormones start to decline more rapidly, we have to look at what type of exercise we are doing and how intense that stimulus is.

As you age, your hormone levels drop. Specifically, male testosterone drops on average 3 percent per year after the age of 40.[5] For women, estrogen peaks in the late twenties and drops 50 percent by the age of 50, with an even sharper decline after menopause.[6] Women as young as 30 will see a minimum of 3–5 percent lean muscle loss per year, and along with this, an increase in body fat and a decrease in bone density.[7] So as we age, we need to increase stimulus that also increases our hormone levels.

The right amount and intensity of stimulus isn't up to you, it's up to your body. The biggest miss by far when people use the adaptation cycle for training is what I call the "intensity gap." They believe they've got the right amount of intensity from the stimulus, even when the body doesn't respond. As I mentioned in Chapter 1 when discussing over-trainers and under-trainers, many people don't get the intended stimulus because there is a gap between what they think they can do and what they can actually do. A study by York University in Toronto took a group of people and put them on a treadmill and asked them to run at a low intensity. Then they were asked to get their heart rate up to 93 percent of max by running at a vigorous pace. Most of the participants thought they were at the 93 percent of max when really they were still well below 75 percent of max heart rate.[8]

When I began working with my friend John, a 53-year-old who had worked out forever, but had never really given it much thought, I quickly realized that he had a large intensity gap. I needed to illustrate this for him, so I asked him to do a step test, where you run on a treadmill and step up the intensity at different increments until you can't go any faster. John came off the treadmill saying he was at max intensity way before he was. Over our next few training sessions I had John use an airdyne bike, on which you use your feet to pedal and your arms to push and pull handles that rotate a fan located where the front wheel would be. The faster you go, the more resistance there is on the fan, and the harder it becomes, but the more power you generate. One day, I asked John to make a bet with me that if he could burn 25 calories in a minute on that bike, he wouldn't have to do 20 burpees in a minute. John didn't think he could do either, but he's the sort of guy who is game for anything, so he took that bet. Because I was next to him, guiding him, cheering for him, supporting him, and because he had something to play for, he hit 25 calories in a minute, almost doubling what he predicted he could do before we started. He was out of breath and his heart was pounding, but he was learning that he was stronger than he thought he was, and this knowledge is what would get him closer to the stimulus he needed to see change in his body. I've done this experiment many different ways with different clients over the years and each time it showed them the gap between what they thought they could do and what they could *actually* do.

Phase 2: Fatigue

Fatigue is the body's response to the stimulus. One of the ways to measure whether we are getting enough intensity with our stimulus is to measure fatigue. The stimulus must have the right intensity to elicit the right amount of fatigue. In order to see adaptation, the stimulus must cause both short-term and longer-term fatigue. Short-term fatigue looks like: "I just ran for two minutes, and now my heart is racing, my legs are burning, and I'm sweating." Longer-term fatigue might last 12–72 hours and occurs after, for example, a group fitness class or bike ride or back squat workout—whatever provides an intense stimulus for your body—and feels like muscle soreness and body fatigue.

Most of us are just moving through our program or our weekly routine without thinking much about this idea of stimulus and fatigue. We think that we will get a training effect just because we showed up and did the thing. The truth is that to see change, we have to know more and do more than just showing up. Some of you may have tried programs, trainers, and gyms that didn't help you make the changes you desired. Most people don't see a failed program as their fault, but rather the program's fault. The coach didn't give me what I needed or the program didn't work for me. That may be true, but it's also worth looking at yourself to see if you are actually doing the work that needs to be done. It comes back to awareness.

My friend Mary learned this the hard way. Mary was new to running and was excited to train for her first half marathon. It wasn't so much about finishing the race, it was about losing weight and feeling better. Once she committed and found an online program she liked, she was on her way. The three-month training plan walked her through a series of weekly long, slow runs; short-sprint intervals; and moderate-range pace running days to prepare her for the half marathon. Much of her training was during Minnesota's late winter and early spring months, which aren't great for outdoor training, so I encouraged her to come to our gym and use our treadmills. I observed that her moderate-range pace runs, which are meant to be run above race pace, and her short-sprint interval runs looked very similar to her long recovery runs. There was very little deviation in her intensity, which in this case was speed. She showed up every day physically, but there wasn't a lot of awareness about why she was doing what she was doing, and after three months of consistent training and following her program, Mary had gained five pounds.

This isn't uncommon, especially among endurance athletes. It's estimated that 78 percent of people who train for a marathon don't lose or gain weight during their training.[9] The reason is because most people don't understand exercise intensity on an individual basis or the importance of exercise intensity as it applies to the way the body adapts. As I stated above, the stimulus must have the right intensity to elicit short- and long-term fatigue. When we don't know what real intensity is or how it feels, the adaptation cycle doesn't work.

In Mary's case, since she thought she had the needed intensity, she also thought she could consume more calories, but her intensity wasn't enough to elicit the change she wanted. Eventually, Mary reached out for help. I didn't have to revamp her plan, I just had to help her understand the adaptation cycle and apply that to the training plan she'd already selected. And even though Mary didn't have a great experience in her first race, she used the knowledge regarding stimulus, intensity, and fatigue to continue training. She ended up losing the weight she had gained and then some, and she ran her second race, which was much more fulfilling. Now she's running all kinds of endurance races. More importantly, by shifting the way she understood fitness, she has been able to see continued improvements and she will be able to work her way through other problems should they arise as she moves forward.

A few questions to ask yourself to see if you are getting the right intensity to cause the appropriate fatigue in your exercise:

1. Do you get out of breath when you train? The type of out of breath where you can't talk and you have to put your hands

on your knees to rest, not all the time, but sometimes? I know this can be scary for some people, like it was for Amy, but you can start slow. Take my mom, for example. She's 85 years old, and she goes for daily walks. There is a hill in her neighborhood, and she tries to walk up it as fast as she can. When she gets to the top she's out of breath, her heart is pounding, her hands are on her knees, and she has to rest. I get the same out of breath when sprinting on the soccer field. We both are getting the right dose of intensity for us individually. The activity is different, but it's appropriate for each of us, and the stimulus elicits the same result: fatigue.

2. Do you feel sore the day or two after a tough training session? Again, this does not need to be after every session, but when you do something challenging, specifically with strength training, the soreness shows you that your body had the right dose of stimulus; it's a form of longer-term fatigue. Note that being sore doesn't always mean you have maximized your body's response. For instance, you can get sore from doing 100 leg extensions in a barre class, but that sore will not elicit the same response that doing dumbbell lunges or back squats or other loaded strength activities will. Heavy-loaded activities tax the central nervous system in a deeper way, causing more fatigue and a greater response. There is a sweet spot for soreness, and sometimes that soreness is delayed after exercise, but it shouldn't last much more than 24–48 hours unless it's an intentional part of your program to overreach, which I discuss in the

ongoing.

Phase 3: Recovery

Recovery is the third step in the adaptation process and is dependent on the first two steps. If you don't have the right stimulus, you won't get fatigued, and thus you really don't need recovery. If you aren't sore and tired after certain training sessions, you didn't get the stimulus your body needed, no matter how much you thought you did. The more intense the stimulus, the greater the fatigue, and the more recovery is needed: "I worked hard, I was sore and tired, I need to recover."

Recovery is any technique to support your body returning to a state ready for another stimulus of intensity. Recovery is just as necessary as the first two phases of the adaptation cycle. It's a balance. If you don't have the appropriate amount of recovery, you will not be ready for the right dose of the next stimulus, as you saw in the case of Linda in Chapter 1. This can lead to injury and burnout. Or you will lower the intensity of your next training to match how you are feeling, and you will not see change and adaptation. Notice in the adaptation graph on page 25 that there are high peaks to show intense stimulus and low valleys to allow for recovery. Learning your timing and cycle will take some patience and some awareness of who you are. The problem for most people, over-trainers and under-trainers alike, is that they never have peaks and valleys in their training cycle, it all sort of just looks the same. They are stuck and will not see the change they are looking for in their fitness.

Note that stress plays a role in how much recovery you need. We have to take life into consideration as we look at stimulus, fatigue, and recovery. Yes, the stress of doing push-ups and sprints is physical stress and affects our fatigue and our readiness to train, but there are other types of stresses that also affect our fatigue and readiness to train. The stress of family, work, kids, finances, and society all affect our fatigue and our ability to train.

When I was the performance coach for Minnesota United FC, in order to see if the players got the right stimulus and fatigue and to know when they were recovered, I measured two key markers every day: heart rate variability and DC output. Heart rate variability (HRV) is the measure of variance between each beat of the heart and shows an athlete's recovery level. DC output is a function of how ready an athlete is to train. It's measured by gathering how much electrical current is in the brain. When the team played a game, the stress on the 11 players who played the most was so great that they needed 48 hours of almost full recovery to be ready to train again. However, the players who didn't play, according to the HRV and DC readiness, were ready to train the day after a game.

One year we had a particularly stressful playoff game that we had to win. It was an away game and the crowd was brutal, with a group of the opposing team's fans sitting behind the bench yelling insults at our players the entire game. Two of our starting players got injured, one got a red card for fighting and was kicked out of the game. The coaches were upset, the players were stressed, and we barely won in overtime. The next day when I measured all 18 players on the team for HRV and DC readiness, I saw that not just the 11 players who played the most needed rest, but all 18 players needed rest, even the ones that didn't get into the game at all. It wasn't because they played a physically demanding game, it was because of the emotional stress of the game. It turned out that everyone needed 48 hours to recover. So know that life stress plays a factor in how hard you can train and how long it will take you to recover.

When most of us think of recovery, we think of a more sedentary lifestyle, like sleeping in, taking naps, or lying on the couch. This isn't the type of recovery I'm talking about. Recovery is active, and in many cases can look like training, but just not as intense. The more we move on our off days, to a certain point, the faster we recover.

Here are five tips that I use and have had clients and athletes use to help with recovery. Remember, we all respond differently, and what's important is to figure out what works best for you.

Sleep

Make sure you are getting a minimum of eight hours of sleep per night. The body simply cannot recover effectively with less than eight hours of sleep. The hormones you seek to force change in your body—testosterone, estrogen, human growth hormone, and other potent anti-aging, muscle-building hormones—are released during the deepest part of your sleep. If you are an efficient sleeper, about 25 percent or about 90 minutes of your total sleep might be deep sleep.[10] So, I recommend a minimum of eight hours of sleep per night. I use an Oura Ring to track my sleep, but other devices can track sleep stages and total sleep. Any decent sleep-tracking device will track heart rate and movement, but you can also follow the tips in Chapter 7 to increase your quality of sleep.

Muscles and Tissue Care

This is probably the most overlooked part of recovery. Caring for muscle and tissue between workouts is key in aiding the body's recovery. Foam rolling supports healthy, supple, and strong tissue and helps with blood flow and recovery. Without this part of recovery, you become brittle, tight, and prone to injury, especially as you age. I like doing most of my mobility—foam rolling and stretching—work before bed because it's a great way to turn the on-switch off and help with sleep. I cover foam rolling in detail in the next chapter.

Collagen and Protein

A collagen supplement can help aid in the recovery process. Collagen is a well-researched supplement, and most studies show that it helps decrease joint pain and increase your ability to recover and feel better after a workout.[11] A 10-gram dose daily is what is recommended. Protein intake, especially once you have a meaningful strength training practice that leaves you sore, is another good way to support recovery. I'll cover more in Chapter 8, but for now, know you will want the right amount and type of protein to effectively support recovery. Protein from animal and/or plant sources is fine. However, animal protein has a higher amino acid profile, which is what helps with muscle recovery. Protein in whole food form has more nutrients and is absorbed better, but powders can also be used to support protein intake. Usually, 1–2 grams of protein per kilogram of body weight is recommended. An easy way to think of this is to have 1–2 palm-sized cuts of lean protein with each meal. I like using hands for portion size because your hand is in proportion to your body size, and you have your hand with you wherever you go. It's not sustainable to always measure and weigh your food.

Hydration

Hydration is one of the most important aspects of recovery and is often overlooked. Drink half of your body weight in ounces of water as a baseline daily. Before you train, have water with a dash of salt or a specific hydration beverage you like. Adding some electrolytes like sodium to your water helps with absorption into the muscle and tissue. As you train, you should sweat; with this sweat, you lose nutrients that must be replaced during and after training. If you are using a sports drink or tablet, make sure the sugars come from glucose or sucrose and watch that the carbohydrates aren't more than 4 percent of the solution. There are a million opinions out there on how you should hydrate. If you are training for a 100-mile race or trying to qualify for the Olympics, it's worth diving deep into the science, but for most of us, just water or water with some added electrolytes is sufficient. You'll need more hydration if you are working out longer than 90 minutes or in extreme heat.

Move!

The best thing you can do for recovery is to move. Walk, swim, bike, but nothing high in intensity or high impact. Just moving gets the lymphatic system working, which will help clear out the soreness. It's okay to do a light workout at maybe 60 percent of the intensity. It's also okay to just try to cover 10,000 steps on a recovery day. Find what works for you, but do not sit around; movement will get you feeling better more quickly.

Phase 4: Adaptation

The adaptation cycle is different for everyone. The stimulus, fatigue, and recovery phases have to be in balance for the full cycle of adaptation to work. The variables (how much intensity and how much recovery, coupled with age, sex, and fitness capacity) will determine what your individual work and recovery cycle looks like. If you are willing to look at your current training through the lens of the adaptation cycle, you'll likely see holes in at least one of the phases. If the stimulus isn't enough, make changes in the type of exercise or the intensity of the activity. If there isn't enough fatigue, add intensity. How much? Until you feel sore and tired the day after a training session. If you don't feel ready to train, add recovery. Understanding the adaptation cycle is half the battle and will help you rebuild or restart your practice in a way that will have more impact now and into the future.

CHAPTER 3

Are You Ready to Train?

Injuries and the Science of Readiness

In the following chapters, I'll be talking a lot about intensity, learning to lift heavy weights, getting out of breath, and making sure that the stimulus is great enough to cause fatigue, but before all this, it's essential to ensure you are ready to train in this way. Before you are able to dive in, you need to make sure you are starting in a place that is right for you. Being ready to train and having the ability to know if your body is ready each day is one of the most important factors in owning your fitness journey. Once you know what your readiness is, it will help you determine not only how hard to work but what type of training is best for you.

Injuries

Injuries can be a major roadblock in training readiness and overall fitness and health. Almost all of us will sustain an injury of some kind in our lives. Understanding why you have an injury or limitations and what you can do to try and solve these problems on your own is a meaningful part of owning your health.

Most injuries that aren't pathological or impact-related are movement-related. This means that the way you are moving or, in some cases, *not* moving can be the root cause of your injury.

When I'm first meeting a new client, we don't sit down in a consult room or go through a series of assessments in front of the gym mirror. We head out on a walk so I can really get to know the person, what they are looking for, what fitness activities they have done and enjoyed in the past, and also what their barriers to fitness are, including what movement-related injuries they might have.

A friend recently came to me because she hadn't been able to run due to an injury. She loved running not only for fitness, but because she ran with a small group of close friends and the community was important to her, as well. She had been injured and unable to run for six months. I'm not a physical therapist, but I also know that, as fitness consumers, by following a few simple practices when it comes to injury prevention and injury recovery, we can take back some of the ownership of our health without having to rely on health care providers for every tweak or pulled muscle we encounter. There is a time and place to use physical therapists, doctors, chiropractors, and other health care providers to help us get out of injury, but before we rely on the healthcare system, we should have some common knowledge about fixing and preventing injury. (Of course, if you try some of these and are not seeing improvement, it's time to see a professional.)

By the time my friend Kate came to see me, she was experiencing pain on the outside of her right foot, which started in her hip. I started Kate on the foam roller, which I use as a diagnostic tool all the time. When I begin to work with a new client, I have them roll on a foam roller everywhere (calves, hamstring, lats, I.T. bands, quadriceps, etc.) to see if any areas are sensitive, which helps me assess tissue health and imbalances and identify what might be problem spots. You should be able to compress any tissue with your body weight without pain. If you can't roll on a foam roller pain-free, the tissue you are compressing is tight and unhealthy. This can be the source of injury or a leading indicator of future injury. I have people roll above and below the injury on a foam roller. Often, they find something sensitive above or below the site of injury, and by compressing that tissue, they desensitize the site of the injury.

The tissue in our bodies around our muscles is connected almost everywhere. It's like grabbing the corner of the bottom of your shirt and pulling on it. You'll notice that it doesn't tighten at the site where you are pulling. Rather, it tightens in the opposite direction or the corner, by your shoulder. By using compression tools like foam rollers, lacrosse balls, tennis balls, or yoga balls for compression in the tissue above or below the site of injury, we can feed relief to the site of injury.

When Kate rolled on the foam roller high on her hip on one side, she could barely handle the compression. This told me something was abnormal. I didn't have to know specifically which muscle was tight or what connective tissue was being affected. All I needed to know was that it meant that something in those spots was not healthy. Once I showed her how to foam roll effectively on those spots, it was easy to determine if it was helping or hurting. She would foam roll for a couple of minutes and then, if she stood up and moved in a way that hurt previously and it now hurt less, we knew that the area she compressed was part of the problem. If it didn't feel better, we knew that the area she compressed was unrelated to her pain. We tested and re-tested different areas above the outside of her foot all the way up to her hip until we could identify a few key spots that seemed to be sensitive to pressure and gave relief after being compressed. The foam roller is a very effective tool for most people in helping with injury and injury prevention. Tips for using a foam roller:

1. There is no wrong way to do it. If there is something you want to compress, find a way to do it. Be creative. You can roll out on the floor or against the wall, as long as you can find ways to get as much body weight on the foam roller as possible.

2. If you are trying to solve a problem or an injury, be open to searching for places above or below the injury site to see if you find something sensitive.

3. "Normal" is full compression of your body weight. This means you should be able to put all your body weight on the foam roller pain-free. (But listen to your body. If you are recovering from an injury or are new to foam rolling, go slow.)

4. Breathe. If you haven't done something like this in a long time, you may be very sensitive to compression. Make sure that you don't hold your breath. Try to breathe deeply into the area you are trying to compress. If you can't take a deep breath, it's too much compression.

5. Pain is okay. If you are working on a troubled spot, it should be painful, but not to the point that you can't breathe. And the pain shouldn't feel weird, like you are causing damage or compressing a nerve, which would feel hot and tingly. It should be a good pain in a way. It should be a very focused experience in which you have to breathe through the tension and pain.

6. When you find a trouble spot, you can just hold there for a trigger-point release.

7. You can also find a spot and then start to move over that spot, pancaking side to side or moving the roller over it with shorter rolls.

8. You can also put pressure on the site and then move the nearest joint to the site you are working on. This is called a tack and floss technique because you are tacking down the unhealthy tissue and then flossing it under pressure as you move the joint. For example, if I'm working on my upper leg or quad, I can find the spot that hurts and then move at the knee by kicking my heel to my butt. This helps the tissue move under pressure, which is a good way to help release it.

Foam rolling can be used for many things, but if you are using it to help with injury or sensitive tissue, it's going to hurt, and that's okay. It may take consistent work on that spot—two minutes per time, several times daily for several weeks—to get sustained relief.

Range of Motion and Stability

Range of motion is how much you can move around a joint. How far can you bend your knee or arch your back? When I talk about stability, I'm talking about the ability to create tightness and torque around a joint. Knowing what level of stability and range of motion are normal in different movements can help you identify where you might be missing either, which is critical to understand before you dive into a new training plan. As we look at different ways throughout the book to assess range of motion and stability, understand that these are related. First, you are only as strong as your weakest link. So, if you are missing 50 percent of your range of motion in a joint, you are risking injury by doing anything outside that range of motion; your body is not used to being in that position and is thus much weaker in that position. This is why at our age we all know someone who went out to play a friendly game of softball in the rec league after not doing anything for 10 years and then sprinted to first base and either pulled a hamstring or ruptured an achilles. This is because they haven't sprinted in a long time and sprinting requires access to a greater range of motion compared to jogging or walking.

With stability comes smoothness and tightness in movement. Not only is this important for performance, but it's important in injury prevention as we look at how to move to do things like lift weights or run faster. When I had Kate, who lacked a strategy for stability, do a squat, her knees wobbled in and out as she moved. When there is stability in the system, there is very little wobble in the joints, but when you are unstable or don't have a strategy to create stability, your body will automatically create it for you, and oftentimes the body doesn't create stability in the best patterns.

Some of these range of motion and stability concepts you can see in everyday movement. If I went to walk and my feet turned out and my knees caved in, I wouldn't look—or be—stable. There is stability in walking with your knees caved in and your toes turned out, but you weren't designed to move in this way; your body just defaulted to it because you were weak or tight in another area. But unless you re-teach yourself good strategies for creating stability, you will get hurt. If you continue to walk or run with your knee collapsing in with each step, eventually the cartilage on the inside of the knee will wear away and this becomes painful and arthritic.

Even small losses in the range of motion or stability can affect you in terms of injury. You might not think it's a big deal if, when you stand, you put more weight on your left foot with your body slightly shifted to the left, but this is your body's way of trying to get out of something tight or weak. Similarly, you might not think a small missing range of motion at your hip is that big of a deal, but when you run a quarter mile, that's about 350 steps, each one bearing your full weight, so over the course of a three-mile run, that's about 4,200 reps on a hip that is missing range of motion, which is going to make your knee hurt.

So, the first step is identifying the problem. That awareness allows you to take a shot at fixing the problem.

Imbalances

Most of us have a dominant and non-dominant side. It's common to be slightly stronger on one side than the other. However, as we develop greater imbalances in muscle tightness, muscle strength, and muscle weakness in opposing muscle groups or from side to side, we increase our risk of injury. Studies show that a 10 percent difference in muscle imbalance can lead to an increased risk of soft tissue injury.[12]

We develop patterns of movement based on how we spend our time during the day. Many athletes have repetitive movement patterns that create imbalances. Soccer players who kick with one foot tend to develop imbalances from one side to the other. Parents who spend all day holding babies on their hips and carrying diaper bags on one shoulder develop imbalances. Sitting hunched over a computer develops imbalances. All of these imbalances increase the risk of injury because they cause our joints to move in sub-optimal patterns to accommodate tightness and weakness. These imbalances also cause a stronger side to do more work than the weaker side, which can lead to overuse injury on the stronger side. When we add stress, like lifting weights or running, to these imbalances, we increase the risk of injury.

One of my clients, who is a professional soccer player, was constantly dealing with a pulled left hamstring. He didn't have any unusual pain when rolling on a foam roller on either leg. But then I had him balance on one leg and do a squat to an 18-inch chair. On his left side, he could squat all the way down to the chair and lightly touch it with his butt and come back up under control. On his right side, however, he would go down about halfway and then just collapse onto the chair.

If you are stronger in your right leg by more than 10 percent and you are doing squats with both feet on the floor, that imbalance can easily be hidden because the strong side will just pick up the slack for the weak side. But he couldn't hide that imbalance doing one-sided squats. He was always pulling his left hamstring, the stronger one, because it was having to make up for all the work that the right hamstring, the weaker one, couldn't do. By doing some simple single-sided activities like hamstring rolls, one-leg step ups, and hip bridges, he was able to gain strength in his weaker side.

Diversifying your practice and finding ways to have single-side activities be part of your regular fitness routine will go a long way as you age and want to avoid injury. Yoga and Pilates are helpful in eliminating side-to-side imbalances. (See Appendix for examples of single-sided exercises to build strength and stability.)

Quick Assessments

The Squat

There are plenty of different assessments that will help you understand where you fit in terms of range of motion and stability, but one of my favorites is to observe yourself squatting in a mirror or on video. I love this as a diagnostic tool because it shows not only what weaknesses and missing ranges you might have but it can also serve as a tool to help you understand the skill of squatting.

Set up your phone in a place where you can see your full body—head to feet—and then record yourself doing 10 squats to a position where the top of your thighs are parallel to the floor, or 90 degrees at the hip and knee. Make sure to record a few squats head on, a few squats from each side, and a few squats from the back view.

What to watch for (and see Appendix for a list of easy fixes):

1. **What is normal range of motion at the knee and hip?** You should be able to squat to parallel at a minimum, meaning your knees and hips should be at 90 degrees and the top of your legs should be horizontal with the floor. If you can't, you may be missing range of motion.

2. **What is normal range of motion at the ankle?** Your toes and heels should be on the floor the entire time. If your heels come up off the floor, you are missing range of motion.

3. **What should it look like when I move through the squat?** You should notice your toes are pointed forward and your knees track slightly outside your feet. There should be no in and out gimbal and wobble at the knee, you should be able to squat up and down smoothly. If you notice your one foot or both are turned out or that your knees move in and out as you squat, you may have a problem creating stability. See Appendix for more information, but know that a simple fix here is to grip the floor with your feet and imagine trying to turn your feet out at the same time as if you are ripping the floor apart. You should feel your glutes fire, thus creating stability.

Arms Overhead

Raising your arms overhead is another important diagnostic tool you can use to see what is weak or tight or what just might not be working. This is a shape we see all the time in the gym and in life: arms go overhead to press something overhead or to do a pull-up. If you play volleyball, the same shape occurs when you block; in tennis, when you serve. When you reach for something on a high shelf at home or go to change a lightbulb in a ceiling fixture you might also have your arms overhead.

To determine if you have a normal range of motion to train overhead, start by lying on your back with your arms by your side with palms facing in. Lock your elbows out so your arms are straight and stiff. Spread your fingertips out as you point through each finger. Now, make sure your legs are tight and knees straight. Take your spine and try to bring your lower back in contact with the ground; this will pull your rib cage in toward your spine and activate your core. Move from your shoulder and slowly bring your arms overhead, keeping elbows locked out, not letting your lower back come off the ground, keeping your ribcage tucked in, and see how far you can go.

What to watch for (quick fixes in the Appendix):

1. **What is normal range of motion?** Normal range of motion is the ability to touch your thumbs to the ground over your head with straight arms while keeping your legs straight and your lower back in contact with the floor.

2. **What if my elbows bend?** Remember the example of pulling on the lower corner of your shirt and it getting tighter in the opposite upper corner by the shoulder? You may have tight tissue. Try rolling on a foam roller on your lats, the muscles that run along your side ribcage, under your arms. Does loosening that tissue allow the shoulder to move better?

3. **What if my lower back comes up off the ground when I raise my arms overhead?** You might need more range of motion in your upper back so you can keep your lower back stable and in place. See the Appendix for how to increase range of motion in the upper back.

If you have an incomplete range of motion and can't get your thumbs to touch the ground overhead in the diagnostic, that's okay. It just means you know your end range of motion and you should work inside that range. But ideally—and this is something you can work toward—you want to have access to your full range of motion in all joints to avoid injury. That's why it's so important to have variety in your training. Play sports, learn new skills, and do things that expose you to a full range of motion.

You don't have to be perfect in order to train. There are a lot of things you can still do even if you are injured or lack stability and range of motion. But you do have to know what is missing so you can train safely.

Hypermobility

If you are very mobile, or hypermobile, you might have access to all of your normal ranges of motion and then some, but there is very little stability as you move, which can also lead to injury. That was my friend Kate's issue. A hypermobile person needs to work on owning positions by showing stability in those positions. Some tension is needed in the system in order to create stability and own those positions. A good place to start is by doing isometric exercises that you hold in one position. For instance, in a squat, you will use your feet to create stability at the hip in a standing position, then squat and hold that bottom position until it burns and you can't hold it anymore, focusing the entire time on using your feet for stability. You can start to work on moving through a range of motion, but you should go slowly to help your body stay connected to the movement.

I describe the feeling you should have as a "grinding" feeling; you are attempting to create some torque and friction. By doing this, you are teaching your brain what it feels like to be stable in a certain position and through the ranges of motion in those positions. Other helpful isometric and slow-moving exercises include planks and wall sits, slow squats and push-ups. But remember that you are not simply hanging out in those positions; you must be active and create stability. (See the Appendix for additional isometric exercises to help you gain stability.)

Balance

Balance is critical as we age. It's also a great way to assess athleticism or loss of athleticism. Balance describes how your brain interacts with your muscles in order to create stability. The older we get, the slower our reaction times are and the less stable we become. This is due to a decrease in lean muscle, range of motion, and proprioception, which is your body's ability to sense movement, action, and location. These three things are critical in having a thriving fitness practice but also in preventing falls as you age.

Before you try these balance assessments, if you have not done any balancing activities for a while or are uncertain of how your balance is, I would recommend starting by standing next to a wall or counter for support in case you lose your balance during the assessment. The first test is simple: just balance on one foot for 30 seconds. If you can do that easily, close your eyes and try the same thing. If still okay, try balancing on one leg, this time with your eyes open, and doing a little lateral jump to see if you can land on the opposite leg, stick the landing, and then hold for five seconds before returning. See if you can do 10 total lateral jumps, sticking the landing each time without letting the non-weight-bearing foot give support.

There are several ways to improve balance. The simplest way to do this is to start using balance daily. In the gym, this means doing exercises while balancing on one foot and using tools like stability balls and BOSU balls in your training. It's also important to remember that if you are outside of the range of motion that you are comfortable with, balance can be very difficult. We see this often in our older population, with falls. If they lack the ability to get up and down off the floor because they don't have the range of motion to get down to the floor, when they lose balance, they just end up falling. Likewise, if you aren't able to create stability when unstable, then balance can be very difficult. Think about the example of using your feet to grip the floor in a squat to help create stability. This is exactly how I coach people to stand on a BOSU ball or a wobble board.

With balance, it is an "if you don't use it, you lose it" scenario. So if your movement practice doesn't involve something like a sport where you have to change direction or jump and land randomly, or if you aren't taking a good yoga class where you have to balance on one foot half the time, you may be out of practice. Simply start by doing what you normally do but on one leg. Do curls on one leg, bench press in a one-leg hip bridge, and brush your teeth on one leg—anything to re-engage with balance and stability. As you learn to create stability in unstable situations, your balance will improve and you will be able to progress to more unstable situations.

Spinal Awareness and Core Stability

Have you ever had a lower back injury? It's different than spraining your ankle. With a sprained ankle you can still get around, you can go to work, do stuff around the house, and sure it might hurt and you have some limitations, but life goes on. Well, not with low back pain. A tweaked low back means you are out, sometimes in bed for days or in pain whenever you move. Making sure you are strong in your core and aware of the shape of your spine in different positions is key in protecting yourself from injury. You can gauge your spinal awareness with a simple hip hinge self-assessment.

To try the hip hinge test, get your phone out again and set it up so you can see your profile view all the way from head to feet. Hit record. One of the keys to this test is to make sure you aren't looking at the video or in a mirror while you are doing the test. Place your feet under your hips and lock your knees out so they are stiff. Put your fingertips behind your ears and point your elbows out. Then fold forward as you hinge at your hip, make sure to keep your knees stiff. Go as far as you can without flexing your spine or rounding your back at all. Hold in what you think is your end range position with your back in neutral for a few seconds and then come back up. You are not testing to see how far forward you can fold, but instead to see how aware you are of the position of your spine. Repeat two or three more times. Now, go grab your phone and review the video.

Could you fold forward and were you aware of what your end range was with a neutral spine or could you have sworn your back was flat but then when you watched the video you noticed that it was rounded? If your back was rounded when you thought it was flat, that can be a problem. It means you have possibly lost touch with your proprioceptive awareness of your back. In other words, you can't feel what your back or spine is doing unless you are looking in a mirror. Most people with loss of spinal awareness are more sedentary and sit for more than half the workday. Several studies show us that sitting is closely related to nerve desensitization.[13] There are detailed recommendations on how to sit less in your day later in the book. But know that anything more than six hours is considered sedentary. A sedentary lifestyle increases the risk of heart disease, diabetes, and obesity, as well as muscular-skeletal injuries like hamstring issues, lower back pain, neck pain, etc. The goal is to sit less than four hours a day.

So, what should you do if you don't have spinal awareness? First, stop sitting so much. Start standing as much as possible. You can slowly work your way into it. Set up your environment at work or home so it can accommodate more standing. I stack books on tables and set up my laptop on top of the books to create my own standing desk. If you work in an environment that doesn't allow for standing, like a truck driver, see if you can get out and walk during breaks. There are some strategic stretches you can also do before you head in to work if you have to sit most of the time (see Appendix). And when not at work, get out and move in as many different ways as possible. Walk, golf, bike...start moving so you have to use your spine in extension, like in an overhead tennis serve. In flexion, like a forward roll. And in rotation, like when you swing a golf club. Even better, start doing yoga. If you want to sit while watching TV, do it on the floor. At first, you might be really uncomfortable, but if you can do it for a few minutes at first and then build your way up, it's a great way to reset your body. According to Healthline, sitting on the floor leads to "natural stability, less hip tension, increased flexibility, increased mobility, and more muscle activity."[14] If you are tight and have a weak core, sitting on the floor will be difficult at first. Don't overdo it. Start with just a couple minutes and then see if you can increase in small increments each day.

If you have pain or are noticing some big issues with these assessments, it's important to first dig into the healing process and be patient. If you have had a movement pattern issue, are missing range of motion, or are unstable and have been like this for years, then it doesn't get fixed overnight. Use a blended approach. Train, get out of breath, work hard at the things that don't affect your injury, but spend time working on the issues causing the pain. Prioritize working on the restrictions you have using the tools I have given you. Physical therapy and other health care options might also be helpful, but know that you do not have to stop training altogether. A blended approach means you are actively working on solving your problems and making good decisions on how to train. Start off slowly, stay away from anything that causes pain. If you have an injured knee and can't run, look at alternatives like biking, running, or swimming for cardio. Sometimes, as we work our way out of injury and we are open to trying new things, we can find new passions in movement.

The Science of Readiness to Train

Now that we have covered some of the assessments you can do to gauge your readiness to train, let's move on to another readiness indicator: the nervous system. The nervous system is a very sensitive part of the human body. It controls many things, like how you breathe, how fast your heart beats, and how you learn. It is also sensitive to physical and emotional stress. By watching how the nervous system responds to exercise, stress, and recovery, we can tell a lot about your fitness level, your ability to recover, what type of training you should do, and how often you should train. In this section, you'll learn how to apply cues from your nervous system to your own fitness.

The central nervous system has two different systems that can help us determine readiness. Both are part of the autonomic nervous system, which is the involuntary part of the nervous system that regulates things like heart rate, breathing, blood pressure, and digestion. The autonomic nervous system is broken down into the parasympathetic nervous system, which is referred to as the rest and digest system, and the sympathetic nervous system, which is responsible for fight or flight. When you are more parasympathetic dominant, your body is rested and ready to train. If you are in a fight or flight state, you are already working and need to let the body recover. If you are in a state of high alert, you might not be ready to train in certain ways. But we are not very often just one or the other; we fall on a scale between rested and high alert.

As I mentioned in Chapter 2, heart rate variability (HRV) is one way to gauge athlete readiness. HRV is the time difference between each beat of the heart. The heart receives a lot of information from the autonomic nervous system, and the way the heart beats and the up and down waves associated with each heartbeat provide an inside view into the autonomic nervous system. An electrical impulse, which comes from the nervous system, controls each heartbeat. We can tell which part of the autonomic nervous system is more engaged based on the variance we see in the difference between beats. The more variance from beat to beat, the more fit and ready you are. The less variance, the less fit and ready you are. In other words, a higher HRV is better than a lower HRV when it comes to readiness to train.

When I work with professional athletes, measuring HRV before training gives me an insight into which players are ready to train hard and which need more rest—objective information that I use as part of a bigger puzzle in determining training patterns. Tracking HRV helps me figure out who can work how hard for how many days in a row and who needs more rest in order to perform optimally and progress. Since we are all different, we all need something different from intensity and recovery.

Tracking readiness for professional athletes is useful, but also an interesting social experiment. What I noticed was the athletes who were very driven and highly motivated to always perform better had a hard time knowing when to rest. These over-trainers thought they were "ready to train" when they often needed rest. The players who were not as driven—under-trainers—often thought they needed a break when they were actually ready to train. For many athletes, it's challenging to look at the objective data and make decisions that go against how they are feeling. What worked was educating them on readiness to train and on what heart rate variability and all other measurables meant. As you'll see in the next chapters, science helps guide us, but the art and connection to how you feel and your ability to be present each day is also critical.

You might not be fighting for a starting spot on a professional sports team, but you *are* fighting for change, for something better, for fitness, and for your health. You don't have to be a professional athlete to know and understand how to gauge training readiness. We all should have some working knowledge of the subject and be able to apply it to our training.

Note that you don't need special equipment, and you don't need a watch or ring, simply a timer. But if you do have a wearable device that tracks your heart rate, note the following in terms of accuracy:

1. An ECG machine is needed to see the full heartbeat wave. Each time the brain sends an electrical signal to the heart, a series of valves open and close to move blood through the chambers of the heart. An ECG can measure each of these contractions in the heart. The full cycle of contractions in the heart consists of a "Q," "R," and "S" contraction. The time difference between a part of this QRS wave compared to the next QRS wave is what is used to gauge HRV. Specifically, the R-to-R wave is used to measure HRV. The full HRV test is done lying down and takes about four minutes to get an accurate reading. The data collected and the time variance between R waves are put into an algorithm that gives a value, often from 1 to 100, showing readiness to train (1 is not ready, and 100 is fully ready).

2. When you use your watch or ring to measure HRV, you do not see a full QRS wave; you just see a beat. When measuring something on a millisecond, it makes a rather big difference to see the R-to-R wave as opposed to the beat-to-beat, which is how your watch or ring measures your HRV since it can't see the full wave like an ECG can. Plus, you are not lying down and keeping still when you measure HRV on your wearable device, which means your heart rate changes as you move, so the time difference between beats might be caused by that movement instead of what the autonomic nervous system is measuring.

3. Still, a wearable device can show you patterns. In other words, you still should be able to see how sleep affects readiness or how fatigue from a previous workout affects readiness. It might not be exact HRV, but it is still measuring beat-to-beat variability, and if tracked over time, you'll notice patterns and be able to make sense of them.

Heart Rate Readiness Warm-up

When people actually see some of the objective information that shows them how hard to train or when to rest, it can be surprising. I challenge you to try this for two weeks once you have started your training program. It's what I call the "heart rate readiness warm-up." I have every athlete and every client do this warm-up every single time they train. It takes two minutes and will give you deep insight into your fitness intensity, capacity, and timing of when you need recovery.

The heart rate readiness warm-up uses the same concept of autonomic nervous system engagement to help determine readiness, which will determine the type of training, how intense the training, and how long the training should be. You have to be open to running the experiment on yourself for at least two weeks while you are training in order to start to see your personal patterns emerge.

1. Find a consistent warm-up element that you can do every time before you train. I like to do a two-minute jog because it's simple.

2. Set your baseline by measuring the distance you cover at your warm-up pace. For example, two minutes equals one lap around the block, or two minutes equals a quarter mile on the treadmill.

3. Measure your heart rate upon completion of the two-minute warm-up. For example, 120 bpm.

4. You have two constants: your two minutes for a jog and the distance: one block or a quarter mile on the treadmill, as examples. You will do that work every single day. Your variable is your heart rate, which will change based on your readiness each day.

5. For example :
    a. Monday 2 mins = .25 mile HR = 120
    b. Tuesday 2 mins = .25 mile HR = 120
    c. Wednesday 2 mins = .25 mile HR = 160

HEART RATE WARM-UP		
	CONSTANT	HEART RATE
Monday	.25 mile jog / 2 minutes	120
Tuesday	.25 mile jog / 2 minutes	120
Wednesday	.25 mile jog / 2 minutes	160

WARNING!!
25% increase in heart rate
for same amount of work

This example tells us that you are not ready to train on Wednesday because your body (heart) is working much harder, 25 percent harder, than it was on Monday, at baseline, to do the same work. Your nervous system is already stressed, so it might be a good day for a walk, a slow run, or maybe it's a day for lighter strength training. I'll put these parts together in various examples later in the book, so you know exactly what's right for you when you see your readiness change.

There are a few things to watch for when running this experiment. If you are working within an intentional overreaching plan, a plan specifically designed to push your body while it is already fatigued in order to force even greater adaptation, it may be okay as part of that plan to train while heart rate readiness is elevated. Your performance might not be as high, but if it's part of the plan, then this is okay temporarily. This is strategic, planned, and very short-term. But if you see your readiness drop drastically (in this case your HR would go up from baseline significantly), you might need to adjust and allow for more rest and recovery.

In some cases, when you keep pushing past an elevated heart rate readiness and other signs of long-term fatigue, such as nagging injury, moodiness, and a low desire to train, your heart rate will simply drop and this means you are beyond short-term overreaching; you could be in the early stages overtraining and adrenal fatigue. This can be dangerous to your health because it can overtax your organs, deplete your hormones, and deteriorate your tissue. Basically, if you don't give your body a rest, your body will refuse to elevate your heart rate; it's protecting you from additional stress in an effort to give itself a rest and keep it protected. Most of us can sustain being pushed while already fatigued for just a few days or up to a week before we need more long-term recovery. This could be 48 hours off or up to five days of active recovery. Once your HR readiness returns to baseline and you feel ready, you'll know it's time to train hard again.

The other thing to watch for is if you are always ready to train. This means that you either aren't working hard enough or you aren't using the right type of training to tax the nervous system. Long, low-intensity cardio and light strength training do not tax the nervous system on a very significant level. Hard intervals that are short and aggressive can tax the nervous system and heavy strength training taxes the nervous system the most. Remember, the key is the hormonal response to what we do for exercise. It's the hormones that elicit change.

Your Feelings Matter

Heart Rate Readiness Warm-up can give you good information, but I also encourage you to align your HR readiness with how you actually feel subjectively. Your feelings are important! This is part of the art that goes into figuring out your fitness program.

To become critical thinkers we need a balance of art and science, which will help you make decisions on what your training should be like each day.

I use these two subjective questions with every client and athlete before a training session. It has helped me teach them about the importance of owning their journey and making decisions that help them excel.

1. On a scale of 1–5, what is my desire to train today? 1=low; 5=high

2. On a scale of 1–5, how sore and fatigued am I today? 1= no soreness/fatigue; 5=very sore/fatigued

Once you have a score, use this chart below to help guide you on how to proceed for the day.

- Desire to train 1 or 2 and soreness/fatigue 4 or 5: Try a walk, some foam rolling, something low impact.
- Desire to train 3 and soreness/fatigue 3: Consider moving but maybe at 60 percent of high intensity.
- Desire to train 4 or 5 and soreness/fatigue 1 or 2: You should be good to redline it and go all out.

Of course, these are just guidelines, but you get the idea. What's important is that you are present and thinking about how you feel, how your body feels, and making decisions for yourself that line up with what is best for you.

A quick reminder that sometimes, after you warm-up, you feel different, and you might change the ratings. You can clear the acidity that causes soreness with a good warm-up and that can, in turn, drive the desire to train. So it's a good idea to ask yourself these questions before and after warm-up.

Once you start to think about how you feel and why you are doing what you are doing, you'll notice patterns in your training. Patterns like, "If I train hard one day, my readiness score doesn't come back up for two days." That's good information, and later in the book you'll learn how to use that to figure out how to progress.

If you aren't ready to train, and you train anyway, then you may be over-training. Or if you are always ready to train, you may be under-training. Dialing this rhythm in is one of the key aspects that takes you from just checking the box on fitness to being an active participant and making decisions about your fitness that will be impactful.

Up next: the truth about strength training!

CHAPTER 4

Strength Training

When you are over 40, you *need* a dedicated strength training practice. Strength training—real strength training—is critical in increasing hormone levels. As your hormones decrease with age, both men and women lose muscle and gain fat. One of the most effective ways to reverse this process is to increase hormone levels through heavy strength training.

There are two big myths about strength training. The first is: "I already do strength training; I do it in yoga or sculpt or barre." Truth: sculpt, yoga, Pilates, and bike boot camp aren't strength training. Neither is using 5 lb dumbbells while riding your Peloton. Sorry! Though these and other forms of exercise that use body weight as resistance are great, the truth is they don't count as strength training and are not helpful at increasing hormone levels.

The second myth of strength training is that it will make you bulky. Again, nope. If you are over 50 years old, you don't have enough anabolic hormones to build muscle—not enough testosterone, estrogen, or human growth hormone. To get bulky you would have to lift very heavy weights—loads you could barely move for more than five reps—almost every day. If you don't know what it's like to do a back squat or deadlift for five to 10 heavy repetitions that feel very heavy, I can promise you that you aren't even close to lifting weights that will make you bulky. And you need at least one year of training to get to a point where you can handle these loads.

Furthermore, to gain muscle to the point of getting bulky, your protein intake would have to be very high to support the recovery needed. Most bodybuilders can't get enough protein to support what they want, so they have to supplement with protein powders. So, you would have to try very hard to achieve that bodybuilder look. With all of this said, women should be able to look bulky if they want. It's part of our culture that says anyone, especially women, can't be attractive if they are bulky. Do what you want to do. Don't buy into what the culture says is attractive. Train the way you want for the outcomes you want.

I have a friend, Keri, with whom I've worked for almost 15 years. No one loves training more than Keri does. She's competitive, supportive, healthy, focused, and fun. But the one thing Keri refused to try over the years, despite the science backing it up, was lifting heavy weights, which she thought would make her bulky. Then, at 48 years old, Keri put on what she called "a layer of fat." Her energy decreased and she noticed her body changing. She spent a couple of years trying to prove that she wasn't going through menopause. She had every test possible, from a Dutch cortisol test, ruling out stress and adrenal fatigue, to iron and ferritin tests, which ruled out an iron deficiency. Finally, when Keri was at the end of her rope, she agreed to develop the skills and work toward lifting heavy weights. After two months on a simple progressive strength program, she shed the "layer of fat" and felt great. She went from a seven-day-a-week training schedule of group fitness, running, and yoga, to three days of dedicated strength work and two days that include cardio sprint intervals and short workouts with bodyweight and kettlebells. Keri is now fitter, leaner, and feels better than ever. She found the right balance for her, and the focus was on heavy strength training. It's different for everyone, but I assure you that weight training should play a part in your plan.

Weight training increases hormone production, which makes you stronger and leaner, increases metabolism, gives you stronger bones, and staves off aging. Remember that we are losing up to 8 percent of our muscle each decade starting at age 30. And at the age of 50 we start losing more bone density than we can produce. Some women can lose up to 20 percent within five to seven years following menopause.[15] It's this loss of lean muscle and bone density that leads to injury, falls, and the inability to be ambulatory.

The only way we naturally see increased hormone production is when the brain is signaled to increase certain sex hormones like testosterone and human growth hormone. This signal comes from the nerves in the muscles asking for more hormones to produce more strength. Each movement you make requires the brain and nerves in your muscles to communicate. When movements are loaded, more nerves are needed and at a deeper level; thus, the brain releases more hormones. This doesn't happen with bodyweight activities such as push-ups because no matter how many push-ups you do, the nerves that the muscle uses to create force only go so deep. When you start to load the same movement with weight, however, you get more muscle nerves engaged on a much deeper level and more hormones are needed to support performance and recovery.

Basics of Strength Training

If you are new to strength training, it will take you some time to learn how to move correctly in order to be able to handle the correct loads you'll need to have the stimulus you are looking for in order to adapt. Keep in mind the following:

Subjective Loading

The best way to know if what you are doing is impactful on a hormonal level is to think of the intensity as subjective rather than objective. Objective loading would be to use a specific weight for a specific activity regardless of how you physically felt. Because we are all different and our bodies need different loads, objective loading doesn't work for most of us. Subjective loading, on the other hand, is based on how you feel. Whenever I have someone do an activity using weights, I have them understand intensity by giving them a description of what it should feel like. For example, if you are doing a set of 10 repetitions, you should feel like the last three reps are very challenging and force you to struggle. You should feel a burn in your muscles, and you should not be able to do five more reps than were prescribed. When you finish the set, you should be out of breath. You should be forced to brace your core, hold your breath, and bear down because you are under pressure and stress. These cues provide context for how intense something should be in order for you to get the stimulus you need.

Focused Multi-Joint Movements

Strength training, real strength training, takes focus. Focus on technique, form, and shape. A good strength training session can be compared to watching a great sporting event. You are focused on everything that is happening, not because you think you have to be, but because you are so into it that you want to be. I can't tell you how many strength training sessions I've observed where people are talking and lifting weights at the same time. It's just not possible to be disengaged and still get to the stimulus that you need.

The menu of strength activities is long and the key is to find the activities that you can do well and then build on those while working on new ones and learning new things. Note that the best strength movements are the ones that you can handle heavier loads because the heavier loads are harder to move and force the body to adapt. Think in terms of multi-joint movements like squats, lunges, step-ups, and presses, as opposed to smaller movements that involve only one joint, such as isolated triceps extensions, leg extensions, and arm curls. The more joints involved in the movement, the more compound, meaning the more muscles are involved and, therefore, the more load you can handle. The body doesn't respond to the movement, it responds to the amount of load you can handle for the movement. So if I do a bicep curl, just flexing at the elbow, you are limited to just using your bicep, one muscle, and one joint, but if you do a squat, you can use your calves, quads, glutes, abdominal muscles, and hamstrings all at once, and your hips, knees, and ankles are all involved in the movement. Therefore you can handle a heavier load in a squat.

The biceps curl max weight is much less than the back squat max weight. Back squat integrates more muscle fibers than biceps curls. It's the response from the load that the central nervous system recognizes and thus responds to with a release of hormones. So you might get sore from doing 100 biceps curls using 5 lbs in the class you just took. That is just muscle soreness rather than central nervous system involvement because you had no deep multi-muscle engagement and no heavy load, thus no hormonal response. Don't get me wrong, there is plenty of room for biceps curls and triceps dips in strength training. As a matter of fact, many of these smaller, more intricate activities can help support overall strength, but really it's the multi-joint compound big movements that are important to start to integrate into your strength practice.

The 100x Rule

If what you are doing for some of your strength cannot be scaled up to be 100 times more intense than what you are currently doing, then it's probably not the strength activity that is going to cause the right amount and type of fatigue. Take, for example, doing side-lying leg raises. You know, the ones that Jane Fonda used to do. You can't scale that up to be 100 times more intense. You could do it faster and you could add an ankle weight, but you cannot add 100 times more intensity. That doesn't mean it's a bad activity; it's actually great to isolate and teach glute activation, but it can't be scaled up very much. On the other hand, if you took dumbbells and held them as you squatted, lunged, or stepped up to a step, you could find a way to progress this movement to make it 100 times heavier. You could move from dumbbells that weighed 10 lbs to a

40 lb kettlebell and then to a barbell that weighed 100 lbs or more. You could start as a beginner doing just bodyweight squats and over time progress to loading a bar on your back that is close to your own body weight or even greater than your body weight. So as you build your strength practice, find movements that have the potential to allow you to move with heavy loads.

Understand Your Body's Limitations

As discussed in the previous chapter, a big part of building your strength practice is being able to identify what issues you might have with movement and range of motion that might lead to injury or restriction down the road. Learning not only how to solve those problems but how to identify a problem before it becomes an injury is important for your awareness and understanding your individual needs. But know that there may be some things you simply can't do in strength training. Not everyone was built to do a full squat, meaning touching their butt to their heels. Can you get better than where you are today? Yes. Does it have to be perfect? No.

Think in terms of risk/reward. Is the reward great enough to outweigh the risk? If not, then don't do it. For example, suppose you are limited in your ability to press things over your head with your arms locked out because you have a shoulder injury or tight muscles. It's not worth the risk to use as heavy a load when you press overhead. Maybe instead you press partially overhead to avoid injury or pain. If you have an old knee injury, maybe squatting isn't your thing, and it may never be your thing, but remember, the body doesn't respond to movement; it responds to load, so if you can't squat, maybe instead you can press with your upper body or do a partial squat. You are not being paid to back squat more than the next guy. If you were, then you may be willing to go closer to that line of risk/reward. But that's not likely. The truth is there is no hurry, no gold medal. We can take our time, focus on form, mechanics, and be aware of how close we are to that line of risk. What's most important is operating inside what you know as safe and effective for you.

Be Willing to Fail

Remember the "intensity gap," how most people can't gauge intensity well? This applies to strength training, as well. I can't tell you how many times in my gym, someone either doesn't know their own strength or they don't believe they can pull the type of intensity needed. It's typical to ask a new client to grab a set of dumbbells and have them estimate how many chest presses they can do with that load. Then once they get started, if I stand over them and encourage them to do more, usually they are off by 50 percent or more. If they think they can do 10, they can often do 20. If you aren't willing to experiment, you might never get the right stimulus to see real adaptation. Knowing our outermost limits is critical for the adaptation cycle. In order to find those outermost limits, you have to be willing to fail; it is the only way to know for sure what your capacity is. Without failure, there is no progression. This might sound intimidating, but it's not. It's exciting. An openness to failing allows potential for growth.

I want you to learn about yourself through fitness, to understand your patterns and how they apply to your health and wellness. Failure in the gym is a great way to practice. The stakes are low. Fitness provides a safe place to practice failure. If you don't run the mile as fast as you wanted or you don't score as high as you planned on the fitness check-up (Chapter 8), you not only get to fail, but you get to see that you'll be okay when you do.

Start Simple

If you are a beginner, it will take about a year of learning, practicing, and experience to develop a strength training practice that is mature and allows you to experiment and be confident. Note that it is worth finding a coach or a solid resource who knows how to coach you in the basics of strength training if you have never done it before. When done correctly, the initial stages of strength training will focus just on simple movements and shapes unloaded and then you will slowly progress to loading these shapes.

It takes about two years to develop a beginning strength practice into something more intermediate that allows you to explore more and feel confident in your ability. This is the point at which you can really start to see changes take place. Of course, if you are a beginner, you'll notice that you are getting stronger quite quickly. You can sometimes see changes in body composition, energy levels, and overall strength in the first six to 12 weeks. But once strength training has been a part of your fitness practice for about two years, you will be able to see significant increases in your strength and you'll be able to start to not only feel more confident in understanding that risk/reward line, but you'll also be able work closer to the heavier loads that provide more impact for you. Just like anything else, when you are starting from scratch, the gains you make are bigger, but at a certain point the incremental gains get harder and require more technique and practice.

I worked with a small group of beginning strength training adults ages 40–50, none of whom had a previous strength training practice. They all had more energy in the first six to eight weeks, everyone had lower body fat percentages within the first six months, and all saw strength increases over the first year, but it wasn't until the second year that they felt confident enough in their form and strength to push through some of the hesitation they had. It was then that they were able to make more significant incremental change. It can take three years or more to become an efficient expert at strength training. The timeline depends on past experiences, genetics, and the quality of training and development. How far you go with this practice depends on your own fitness goals.

In the following chapters I will outline a system that will help you understand how to move, starting from simple and progressing to complex. And I hope you will embrace real strength training the way I've seen so many of my clients do.

CHAPTER 5
Fitness Check-up

When I was in college, in order to make the soccer team, we had to pass a fitness test that consisted of running three miles in less than 18 minutes. The test always took place at 5:00 AM on the first day of preseason training. The course was through a hilly neighborhood in Des Moines, Iowa, next to the Drake University campus. Our coach made it clear: If you didn't pass the test, you would get cut from the team. I was a midfielder and my job was to run all over the field, so running three miles in less than 18 minutes wasn't hard for me back then. But the goalkeepers, whose positions don't require a lot of running, also had to run the course that fast. I couldn't help thinking that the coach should have different time requirements based on position. After all, the data existed, even back then, showing how much distance an average player in each position covered in a game. If the coach's goal was to ensure that each player was fit enough to effectively do his job, he should have looked into the standards for each position and tested us on those. When I asked about the reason behind the 18 minutes, he said, "It's always been that way." Similarly, industry fitness standards often are not applicable because they don't take into account age, sex, and where you, specifically, are right now with your fitness. That's where the fitness check-up comes in.

Regular fitness check-ups are just as important, if not more important in terms of prevention, as regular medical check-ups. A fitness check-up is a series of fitness assessments and the specific standards that go along with them that will help you understand how to compare yourself to others of your age and sex who are healthy, strong, and fit. These assessments will give you insight into your overall fitness capacity and also help you know where to start your training and what the right progression is for you.

I've gathered the data so you can see how you stack up against what is normal and healthy for someone your age and sex. The key to creating fitness standards is finding the right data that supports realistic performance and is representative of strong correlations between fitness, longevity, and health. You will not be comparing yourself to Olympic athletes 25 years younger than you, nor will you be comparing yourself to hardcore fitness enthusiasts who live, breathe, and eat fitness—people like Paula Ivan, a 60-year-old female who ran a 4:15 mile, or Carlton Williams, a 50-year-old man who did 2,220 push-ups in 60 minutes. Instead, we will use standards that represent the best possible outcomes attainable given your age, sex, and busy lifestyle.

The data I've based these fitness standards on comes from a range of studies and real experiences with millions of participants. I've selected five assessments that provide a wide range of cardio and strength standards as well as mobility and stability standards. These standards are relatable, well-researched, and designed to help you take some simple steps to get closer to where you want to be with your fitness. These assessments will give you insight into your overall fitness capacity. After doing the tests and seeing where you fit within the standards, you will have a Fit Score that shows your overall fitness and will give you a clear starting place.

Note: these tests don't define you. I know what it's like to feel stressed about doing fitness and health tests. When I am healthy, fit, and thriving, I find myself excited about trying to beat my old scores to make sure I'm getting better. But when I am not in a good place with my fitness, it can be intimidating to see how far I have fallen from my peak fitness. I have to remind myself that my fitness check-up is a tool that will help me get unstuck and move forward with my fitness goals again. The following have helped me get through health and fitness check-ups:

1. **The results don't define me.** It helps me to see these assessments and results as tools that help me tailor a program to meet my specific needs. I know how important it is to have an individualized program designed to meet me where I'm at physically and emotionally. Seventy-three percent of people who start a fitness program quit because the program is too challenging, boring, or ineffective.[16] Understanding where you are today and setting up the right starting point is crucial.

2. **Don't obsess over your score.** The healthiest place for these fitness numbers to live is in the background, as a tool that we can look at once in a while for guidance. If these numbers drift to the foreground and cause too much stress, they no longer serve their purpose and they steal from connection, internal drive, and joy. You might need to remind yourself to keep the focus on the work that you are doing and how you feel rather than on your Fit Score.

3. **Stress can be good if used correctly.** When I do my fitness check-up, I sometimes feel stressed, but I remind myself that it's part of the process. The stress shows that I care and am passionate about my health. Once I recognize that, I have awareness and feel more in control.

4. **Efficacy!** As much as I celebrate blue ribbons and gold medals for everybody, I know that when it comes to using fitness as an indicator of health, we need to have objective data that shows us whether what we are doing is working or not, thus giving us the information we need to ask questions and make adjustments. We aren't always going to win or see the results we want, but I'd rather have the truth so I know how to move forward effectively.

Most fitness assessment studies are done in a clinical setting, requiring blood panels, gas exchange data, and sometimes muscle biopsies. Those kinds of assessments would be very challenging, if not impossible, to replicate at home or even in a gym. Instead, the following assessments come from studies of healthy, active, and thriving populations across the world. They are basic, simple to follow, and can be done in your home without equipment. The magic is in the standards associated with each test. The standards stand for something concrete in each assessment. For example, I want you to walk away knowing exactly what having more upper body strength means and why you need it as opposed to just trying to improve upper body strength. How much improvement? What is the point of the goal? What benefits will I see? The standards give you something real to understand, compare, and chase.

These five tests will give you an overall view of your fitness. Each test is different and will test a different aspect of your fitness. Remember, it's the broader view of fitness that counts here. Doing well across all disciplines counts more than doing great in one discipline. For each test, there is a performance score from 0 to 5 based on the standards for each test. When added up across all five tests, your total score will be your Fit Score. This score will give you a picture of your overall fitness level and provide you with a specific starting point. Before I explain each of the tests, here are the most frequently asked questions:

What if I can't do one of the tests?

If you can't complete a test due to injury or restriction, don't worry. There are alternatives for some of the assessments designed to test the same physical markers but in a different way. If the alternative doesn't work for you and your restriction or injury inhibits you from doing the type of movement required for the test, that's also okay. You can skip the test you are unable to complete and think about coming back to it once you are able. It will be helpful, however, to consider why you cannot do the test and investigate what restricts you, as discussed in Chapter 3. But know that none of the assessments will ask you to do anything that is not part of what is a normal range of motion or normal strength. If you can't squat because your knee hurts, then you should know why and be able to take a pass at how to fix it. After all, it's your knee, and being healthy requires a certain level of awareness. Too often, we dismiss the reasons behind our physical limitations. Take the steps now to figure out what is causing pain or lack of range of motion, etc. So, it's okay to move past an assessment if pain is involved, but ignoring that pain isn't a solution. If you have to skip a test to attain an overall Fit Score, you can take the average of the tests you could complete and apply that to the tests you could not.

What order should I do the tests in, and how much do I rest between each test?

The order of the tests is important because you want to score accurately for your fitness level for each test. Going from strength to endurance will give you the best expression of your fitness capabilities in each domain. I recommend this order: 1) Longevity Predictor Sit-to-Rise-Off-the-Floor Test; 2) All-Cause Mortality Grip-Strength Test; 3) Swiss 1-Minute Sit-to-Stand Test; 4) Air Force 2-Minute Hand-Release Push-ups, and 5) Endurance 1-Mile Time Trial. Make sure you are warmed up before you test.

Recovery: Make sure you are fully recovered between each test. Minimum rest should be three minutes; maximum rest can be whatever you need. Pay attention to how you feel. You should feel completely rested before moving on to the next test. Make a note of how much rest you need between tests so that when you come back to retest, you can accurately compare your scores.

What if I don't even test on the scale as a beginner?

That's okay, you're not alone. Remember, the standards are set by a population of fit, active people. You don't have to be there today, but the goal is to work toward a place where your fitness check-up meets the standards. But everybody has to start somewhere. And knowing where you are will help guide your fitness program.

Warm-up

Before you try any of the assessments, make sure you are warmed up. Below is a general warm-up, but if you have a different warm-up that works for you, go ahead and use that. The goal of the warm-up is to make sure you have reviewed all the shapes represented in the assessments and that your muscles and body temperature are warm.

Step 1: Pick up

Walk, bike, jog, or do any cardio movement for six minutes. Each minute, pick up your intensity so you are slightly out of breath at the end and have to focus on what you are doing.

Step 2: Plank to Push-up

Start in a high plank position and hold for a five-second count, then lower your body to the floor while keeping your shoulders and hips connected and aligned. Once on the floor, push your body weight back up to keep the same shoulder and hip alignment. You can also do this with your knees on the floor. Do 3–5 repetitions.

Step 3: Squat Prep

Stand with your feet slightly wider than shoulder-width apart. While keeping your heels and toes on the ground, with your toes pointing forward, squat down and drive your knees out laterally as your feet grip the floor. Touch your butt to a surface 18 inches from the ground. Do 5–10 repetitions. If you can't do this, use a wall to do a wall sit, holding for 10–30 seconds at the 18-inch mark.

Step 4: Get Ready

If there is anything you need to do to get ready, add that. Stretch anything you need to stretch. Practice anything you need to practice. Your first test should start five minutes from the end of your warm-up.

The Assessments

1) Longevity Predictor Sit-to-Rise Off the Floor

Why this test?

The Sit-to-Rise test is a creative way to gauge more than one aspect of fitness. Range of motion, mobility around joints, and your ability to have flexion, extension, and rotation in your body are what lay the groundwork for developing a sustainable fitness and strength practice. This assessment tests stability, balance, strength, and mobility, all skills that can sometimes be overlooked when testing for fitness capacity. These skills are necessary not only to develop a deeper fitness level and prevent injury, but the research around the ability to sit on the floor and stand up using no hands shows a strong correlation to longevity.

Purpose:

Test strength, mobility, balance, and stability.

History and research:

In 2012, a Brazilian team of researchers led by Dr. Claudio Gil Araujo published a Sit-to-Rise study in the *European Journal of Cardiovascular Prevention*. In their study, 2,000 people ages 50–80 were asked to perform the Sit-to-Rise test. All participants were followed for six years. One hundred fifty-nine of the 2,000 participants died during those six years, and out of those, only two had passed the Sit-to-Rise test.[17] From this study, we can draw a correlation between longevity and the skill of sitting on the floor and rising without the assistance of hands and other appendages and joints. Being able to sit and rise with no hands does not mean you will live to be 100, of course, but I am convinced that this research adds a lot to your Fit Score and the breadth and scope of how you need to start to look at your fitness. This test requires more than a single element of fitness and it's functional because it is a way of getting up and down off the ground, which becomes a very important skill as we age.

Pros:

Easy to understand. Any flat surface will work.

Cons:

More challenging than it seems.

Protocol:

Start standing and lower yourself to the ground in a crisscross position. To score 5 points, you cannot use your hands, arms, knees, or sides of your legs. Then, stand back up the same way for another 5 points. You get a 1-point deduction for each appendage or joint with which you touch the ground.

What to watch out for:

Please make sure you are warmed up before doing this test.

How to Score:

- 5 points for sitting without using hands, arms, knees, or the side of your legs.
- 5 points for standing back up in the same way.
- 1 point deduction for each appendage or joint you touch the ground with.

Alternative:

None

2) All-Cause Mortality Grip-Strength Test

Why this test?

Grip strength is not only a reflection of overall strength, but research shows that it is also closely tied to longevity. A study by Dr. Mark Pederson, published in the National Library of Medicine in 2023, measured DNA age acceleration in conjunction with grip strength. DNA age acceleration is a way to measure your DNA to see if it matches your chronological age. The study found that those with below-average grip strength had accelerated DNA, meaning their DNA was showing that they were older than they actually were.[18]

For 25 years, the way that I have been testing and recording grip strength is by having my clients dead hang from a bar. The dead hang test considers more than just grip strength; it considers body weight to grip strength ratio as you will be asked to hold your body weight from a bar.

Purpose:
Test grip strength.

History and research:
Most grip strength studies use a hydraulic hand dynamometer, but it's not practical to expect everyone to be able to access that kind of tool. The dead hang doesn't have much clinical research history, so I've had to rely on my experience and the experiences I've found in communities that are thriving, healthy, and strong at our age. Since there is little data on standards for the dead hang, you'll notice that I have adjusted the age-predicted dead hang times. I did this based on a study from the National Library of Medicine in which 1,710 subjects' grip strength was measured from the age of before 50 to over 65 years old. The community that took part in the study was from Tobago and had above-average hand-grip strength due to the amount of physical activity in their daily lives. Up to age 50, participants gained grip strength, and then at the age of 50, every 4.5 years they lost 2.2 percent of their grip strength up to the age of 65, at which point there was a 3.8 percent loss every 4.5 years.[19] I

am using a 2.2 percent deduction in your standards for each age bracket. You will also note in the charts that men and women have different standards. In most studies, men have a stronger grip strength than women when using a dynamometer. In a study published in the National Library of Medicine in 2022, men averaged a grip force of 48 kg while women averaged 33 kg.[20] I have applied that difference to the scoring chart for dead hang standards.

Pros:

This test is not technical at all. Find a bar from which your feet don't touch the ground and hang as long as possible.

Cons:

Finding a bar to hang where your feet can't touch the ground may be challenging for those who don't belong to a gym or have access to playground equipment.

Protocol:

1. Using an overhand grip, hang from a bar where your feet don't touch the ground. Start a timer.
2. Hang as long as possible. You can release your grip once you can no longer hang from the bar. Stop the timer.

What to watch for:

If the bar is too high to jump to, you can use a step to get the bar.

How to Score:

See chart for your age and sex in Chapter 6.

3) Swiss 1-Minute Sit-to-Stand Test

Why this test?

In Switzerland, one of the top four countries for life expectancy, 74 percent of the population from 35 to 64 years of age is active. The government has implemented an in-depth plan around physical activity and tracks it closely, so it's a great resource for fitness data. The fitness culture involves hiking, running, biking, and skiing. The government promotes movement at a young age by not busing kids to schools. Rather, students walk to and from school, high-lighting the priority of lifestyle and health.[21]

Purpose:

Test lower body strength endurance.

History and Research:

Muscle strength endurance is among the most important indicators of current health and longevity predictors in healthy individuals and people with chronic disease. The Swiss Sit-to-Stand Study, performed in 2013 with over 7,000 participants, was part of a national campaign to understand the correlation between lower body strength endurance and overall health.[22] The Swiss health statistics are some of the best in the world, but this particular test bases the standards on some very specific numbers. The test clearly shows decreased lower body strength endurance result in an increased risk of mortality. In another study related to lower body strength endurance, those with above average lower body strength endurance had a 14 percent lower risk of death.[23] In the Swiss Sit-to-Stand Study, the median score was 50 Sit-to-Stands in one minute across all ages. The study concludes that below-average scores, calculated at the 25th percentile or less, indicate a higher risk for disease and increased health risks.

Pros:

Easy to do, not much equipment required, just a chair or bench that is 18 inches high.

Cons:

If you have a lower-body injury that restricts you from doing squats or sitting down and standing up rapidly, this might not work for you. In which case, see the alternative test.

Protocol:

1. Start standing with your knees and hips fully extended.
2. Your feet should be right outside your hips.
3. Squat to touch your butt to a bench, box, or chair 18" from the floor.
4. Hands are by the side or on hips; don't put hands on legs to support.
5. Stand back up to the start position and repeat as many times in one minute as possible.

What to watch for: Make sure you touch your butt to the 18-inch bench and stand all the way up each time.

How to Score:

See chart for your age and sex in Chapter 6.

Alternative:

Wall Sit

See chart for your age and sex in Chapter 6.

4) Air Force 2-minute Hand-Release Push-up Test

Why this test?

Upper body strength is important for a number of reasons, but according to a 44-year study on over 2,000 people published in the National Library of Medicine, those with better upper body strength live longer and have later onset of disease.[24] The hand-release push-up assures that your body goes all the way to the ground with each push-up, thus giving the data more accuracy.

Purpose:

Test upper body strength endurance.

History and research:

It's easy to cheat when doing a push-up and challenging to see how low or high participants go on each push-up, making the data unreliable. But in January 2022, the U.S. Air Force released its new physical fitness test standards, which included a 2-minute hand-release push-up test.[25] The U.S. Air Force takes its fitness seriously. I don't mean that they have crushing fitness assessments that are impossible to pass, but rather that they are serious about finding the right way to measure and progress their population. In

2021, general Charles Q. Brown Jr. said, "We are moving away from a one-size-fits-all model." They view fitness as a tool for health and are working on creating an inclusive, well-rounded approach to engage their entire community.[26] It's working. A recent report by the Rand Corporation found that less than 1 percent of U.S. airmen and airwomen are at risk of adverse health conditions, and every single marker in their fitness tests is headed in the right direction.[27] The hand-release push-up test that they adopted assures that everyone covers the same distance in each repetition. This is the most valid upper body strength endurance test with the biggest pool of data points that I have found. I have made a few minor adjustments to the women's scoring because only 20 percent of the air force is made up of women pilots and officers,[28] so I wanted to broaden the pool a bit, and I did this by conducting the hand-release push-up test on over 1,000 healthy active adults.

Pros:
The data is more accurate because participants will have to do a full push-up, touching the chest to the floor.

Cons:
Like any other test, if form and guidelines are not followed, the results can be skewed. Fatigue can also lead to poor execution of the movement.

What to watch for:

Make sure that your body moves as one unit once you release your hand from the ground and push your way back up. Don't worm your way up.

Protocol:

These are the exact instructions used by the Air Force:

1. Hands flat on ground.
2. Push the body up as a single unit to fully extend elbows.
3. Bend elbows to lower your body down to the ground. The chest and thighs hit the ground at the same time.
4. Once you are on the ground you must fully extend your arms from the ground making sure you have a 90-degree angle from arm to trunk.
5. Return arms to the start position and repeat.
6. Resting can only be done in the up position.
7. You have 2 minutes to complete as many hand-release push-ups as possible.
8. If you rest on the floor and not in the up position, the test will be terminated and your score to that point will be recorded.

How to Score:

See the chart for your age and sex in Chapter 6. Scale down if you can't complete 1 rep or more of a full hand-release push-up. In which case a bent knee push-up would be just fine. Remember, part of the goal is to create efficacy around our fitness practice, and using the fitness check-up gives you the opportunity to always come back to where you started to see if you are improving. Yes, it's nice to see what fit and healthy standards are, but understanding the importance of making this work for you is more important than following strict guidelines.

Alternative: High Plank Hold
See the chart for your age and sex in Chapter 6.

5) Endurance 1-Mile Time Trial
Why this test?
This test has more up-to-date standards than most cardiovascular endurance tests and it's very easy to execute. Even if you can't run the entire time, you can cover the mile doing run/walk intervals. To make this even more concrete, the research shows us how significant cardiovascular health is as a predictor of heart disease. A 55-year-old man or woman who can cover a mile in 15 minutes has a 30 percent chance of developing heart disease. However, a 55-year-old man or woman who can run a mile in eight minutes has a 10 percent risk of developing heart disease.[29]

Purpose:
Test cardiovascular endurance.

History:
Accurate times for the mile have been recorded since 1850. In 1886, Walter George set the first official record for the mile at 4 minutes, 12 seconds. I am, of course, not expecting you to run anywhere near that fast! I use data from Running Level, a website that allows anyone to input their running performance's best results

for specific distances. The site has millions of data points from users who have posted their mile times. Each month, more than 200,000 people post times. All results are broken down into norms based on age and sex.[30] When I look at the results they post, they line up with what I see as valid based on my years of experience in fitness. Our fitness check-up uses Running Level normative data for the endurance 1-mile time trial.

Pros:
Easy to do. Find a local track, use a treadmill, or measure a mile using a GPS tracker on your phone.

Cons:
It can be challenging if you haven't done this in a while.

Protocol:
1. Warm-up according to the guidelines.
2. Run one mile, timed.

Strategy:
Depending on what feels right, you can either go out fast or be steady and try to finish strong. Feel your way through it and do what is right for you. There is no right or wrong way to attack this.

What to watch for:
If you are not running on a track or a treadmill, be sure that the course you pick is as flat as possible.

How to Score:

See the chart for your age and sex in Chapter 6.

Alternative:

2,000 meter row

After you have completed your fitness check-up, look through the charts in Chapter 6 to help you identify your Fit Score. The charts are separated by age and sex. Remember, as you compare your scores to the ones you will see in the chart, be mindful that these norms are set by active, healthy, thriving communities that I know to be the right balance of sustainable, realistic fitness.

If you blew past these fitness check-up assessments with no problem or if you want more of a challenge, see the Appendix for my three higher-level fitness tests.

CHAPTER 6
Your Fit Score

Fitness Check-up Standards Fit Score

If you are nonbinary, choose the category with which you feel most comfortable.

MEN | 40-45					
Points	**1**	**2**	**3**	**4**	**5**
Test	**Beginner**	**Novice**	**Intermediate**	**Advanced**	**Elite**
Endurance 1 Mile Time Trial	9:06 - 8:23	8:22 - 7:07	7:06 - 6:12	6:11 - 5:32	5:31>
Air Force 2 Minute HR Push Up	28-32	33-37	38-42	43-47	48+
Swiss 1 Minute Sit to Stand	25-36	37-44	45-52	53-68	69+
All Cause Mortality Sit to Rise	0	1-3	4-6	7-9	10
Longevity Predictor Dead Hang	10-30 seconds	31-60 seconds	61-90 seconds	91-120 seconds	121+ seconds

WOMEN | 40-45

Points	1	2	3	4	5
Test	Beginner	Novice	Intermediate	Advanced	Elite
Endurance 1 Mile Time Trial	9:26 - 11:09	8:06 - 9:25	7:07 - 8:05	6:23 - 7:06	6:22>
Air Force 2 Minute HR Push Up	14-18	19-23	24-28	29-33	34+
Swiss 1 Minute Sit to Stand	26-34	35-40	41-47	48-64	65+
All Cause Mortality Sit to Rise	0	1-3	4-6	7-9	10
Longevity Predictor Dead Hang	7-20 seconds	21-40 seconds	41-60 seconds	61-80 seconds	81+ seconds

MEN | 46-50

Points	1	2	3	4	5
Test	Beginner	Novice	Intermediate	Advanced	Elite
Endurance 1 Mile Time Trial	8:42 - 10:54	7:22 - 8:41	6:26 - 7:21	5:44 - 6:25	5:43>
Air Force 2 Minute HR Push Up	22-26	27-31	32-36	37-41	42+
Swiss 1 Minute Sit to Stand	25-34	35-43	44-51	52-69	70+
All Cause Mortality Sit to Rise	0	1-3	4-6	7-9	10
Longevity Predictor Dead Hang	10-29 seconds	30-59 seconds	60-88 seconds	89-117 seconds	118+ seconds

WOMEN | 46-50

Points	1	2	3	4	5
Test	**Beginner**	**Novice**	**Intermediate**	**Advanced**	**Elite**
Endurance 1 Mile Time Trial	9:50 - 11:38	8:28 - 9:49	7:26 - 8:27	6:40 - 7:25	6:39>
Air Force 2 Minute HR Push Up	13-17	18-22	23-27	28-31	32+
Swiss 1 Minute Sit to Stand	25-34	35-40	41-49	50-62	63+
All Cause Mortality Sit to Rise	0	1-3	4-6	7-9	10
Longevity Predictor Dead Hang	7-20 seconds	21-40 seconds	41-59 seconds	60-78 seconds	79+ seconds

MEN | 51-55

Points	1	2	3	4	5
Test	**Beginner**	**Novice**	**Intermediate**	**Advanced**	**Elite**
Endurance 1 Mile Time Trial	9:03 - 10:54	7:41 - 9:02	6:41 - 7:40	5:58 - 6:40	5:57>
Air Force 2 Minute HR Push Up	22-26	27-31	32-34	35-39	40+
Swiss 1 Minute Sit to Stand	24-34	35-41	42-52	53-68	67+
All Cause Mortality Sit to Rise	0	1-3	4-6	7-9	10
Longevity Predictor Dead Hang	9-28 seconds	29-58 seconds	59-86 seconds	87-114 seconds	115+ seconds

WOMEN	51-55				
Points	**1**	**2**	**3**	**4**	**5**
Test	**Beginner**	**Novice**	**Intermediate**	**Advanced**	**Elite**
Endurance 1 Mile Time Trial	12:16 -10:22	10:21- 8:55	8:54 - 7:50	7:49 - 7:01	7:00>
Air Force 2 Minute HR Push Up	10-14	15-19	20-24	25-29	30+
Swiss 1 Minute Sit to Stand	23-32	33-38	39-46	47-59	60+
All Cause Mortality Sit to Rise	0	1-3	4-6	7-9	10
Longevity Predictor Dead Hang	6-19 seconds	20-39 seconds	40-58 seconds	59-76 seconds	77+ seconds

MEN	56-60				
Points	**1**	**2**	**3**	**4**	**5**
Test	**Beginner**	**Novice**	**Intermediate**	**Advanced**	**Elite**
Endurance 1 Mile Time Trial	11:22 - 9:24	9:23 - 8:02	8:01 - 6:58	6:57 - 6:13	6:12>
Air Force 2 Minute HR Push Up	21-25	26-30	31-33	34-38	39+
Swiss 1 Minute Sit to Stand	22-32	33-40	41-47	48-62	63+
All Cause Mortality Sit to Rise	0	1-3	4-6	7-9	10
Longevity Predictor Dead Hang	9-27 seconds	28-57 seconds	58-84 seconds	85-111 seconds	112+ seconds

WOMEN | 56-60

Points	1	2	3	4	5
Test	**Beginner**	**Novice**	**Intermediate**	**Advanced**	**Elite**
Endurance 1 Mile Time Trial	10:59 - 13:00	9:27 -10:58	8:18 - 9:26	7:26 - 8:17	7:25>
Air Force 2 Minute HR Push Up	9-13	14-18	19-23	24-28	29+
Swiss 1 Minute Sit to Stand	21-29	30-35	36-42	43-60	61+
All Cause Mortality Sit to Rise	0	1-3	4-6	7-9	10
Longevity Predictor Dead Hang	6-18 seconds	19-38 seconds	39-50 seconds	51-74 seconds	75+ seconds

Alternative Assessments
Wall Sit Test[31]
(The data from this test doesn't break down by age group but still gives us some general ideas of what is possible.)

WALL SIT TEST			
Rating	Points	Males (seconds)	Females (seconds)
Elite	5	>100	> 60
Advanced	4	75-100	45-60
Intermediate	3	50-75	35-45
Novice	2	25-50	20-35
Beginner	1	< 25	< 20

Plank Hold[32]
(The data provided does not differentiate by sex or age, but again it gives us a good understanding of what healthy, active adults are capable of.)

PLANK HOLD		
Rating	Points	Time
Elite	5	> 6 minutes
Advanced	4	4-6 minutes
Intermediate	3	2-4 minutes
Novice	2	1-2 minutes
Beginner	1	30-60 seconds

2K Row[33]

2 KILOMETER ROW					
MEN	**1**	**2**	**3**	**4**	**5**
Age	**Beginner**	**Novice**	**Intermediate**	**Advanced**	**Elite**
40-45	8:23 -7:52	7:51-7:20	7:19-6:50	6:49-6:22	6:23>
46-50	8:33 -7:59	8:00-7:29	7:28-6:58	6:57-6:31	6:30>
51-55	8:43 - 8:11	8:10-7:37	7:36-7:06	7:05-6:39	6:38>
55-60	8:59 - 8:25	8:24-7:51	7:50-7:19	7:18-6:51	6:50>
Women					
Age	**Beginner**	**Novice**	**Intermediate**	**Advanced**	**Elite**
40-45	9:56 -10:51	9:00 - 9:55	8:13 - 9:01	7:30 - 8:12	7:29.6>
46-50	10:02-10:58	9:08-10:01	8:18 - 9:07	7:35-8:17	7:34.5>
51-55	10:09-11:05	9:14-10:08	8:23-9:13	7:40-8:22	7:39>
55-60	10:28-11:26	9:31-10:27	8:39-9:30	7:54-8:38	7:53>

Once you have completed your fitness assessments, add the points from each column based on your results. This will give you a Fit Score. Your Fit Score will help you identify a program to follow in Chapter 8.

FIT SCORE	
Rating	Score
Elite	23-25
Advanced	19 - 22
Intermediate	15 - 18
Novice	11 - 14
Beginner	0 - 10

I have also included this tracking chart so you can continue to come back to your Fit Score as you progress to see what's working for you and what changes need to be made. Depending on what feels right for you, retesting can be done every month or once a year. If you are just starting, it might be nicer to track things at closer time intervals as you are more likely to see change. However, as you progress, improvements in your Fit Score will take more time, so less frequent testing is what I recommend.

MY PROGRESS CHART

Assessment	Date / Pts. / Time	Date / Pts. / Time	Date / Pts. / Time	Date / Pts. / Time	Date / Pts. / Time	Date / Pts. / Time	Date / Pts. / Time
Endurance 1 mile Time Trial							
Air Force 2 Minute HR Push Up							
Swiss 1 Minute Sit to Stand							
All Cause Mortality sit to rise							
Longevity Predictor Dead Hang							

CHAPTER 7

Lifestyle and Nutrition

Before we move into fitness plan examples based on Fit Scores, let's talk lifestyle and nutrition. I've come to realize over the last two decades that fitness, *real* fitness, is not about how much you can bench press or how many squats you can do; it's about longevity and survival. The type of fitness associated with longevity and survival is real, functional fitness. It's broad, inclusive, and diverse. It isn't measured by your mile pace or calories burned. It's measured in how long you live and your quality of life. Of course, the fitness we gain in the gym or on the bike or following our favorite app are important and support longevity and survival, but there is so much more.

My good friend and client Ethan Zohn, winner of CBS's *Survivor: Africa*, taught me this lesson the hard way. I helped Ethan prepare for many of his extreme adventures, including the 2019 *Survivor: Winners at War*, the 40th season, which featured 20 past winners. It took almost a year to get Ethan, who is also a two-time cancer survivor, to a place where he was happy with his fitness level. We spent time online together and we ran training camps in Minneapolis, on his farm in New Hampshire, and at his summer house, which was outside of Atlanta at the time. As we approached the filming and competition date, I put together a five-day, winner-takes-all training camp as close to a real "survivor" experience as I could come up with. I was stronger, faster, leaner, and more athletic than Ethan; after all, I spent my days in the gym, and my life revolved around health and fitness. Ethan was coming off of two major battles with cancer and his job was traveling the world as a public speaker sharing his story. I thought I could beat him.

The five-day camp was full of fitness challenges, solving puzzles, throwing knives at targets, living in the woods, making fire, and swimming through lakes, all on limited calories. It didn't take long for me to realize that fitness wasn't just about how far I could run or how much weight I could lift; it was about how I applied my skills in real-life situations. Well, I didn't win a single point, and if it had been a real *Survivor* season, I definitely would have been voted off after the first day. I specifically remember one challenge: we had to hold a heavy medicine ball over our head as we made our way through a series of balance beams we made out of 2 x 4 boards that rested on uneven tree stumps in the forest. I had no problem holding something heavy over my head and I could do anything in the gym while I balanced on one foot (one-leg squats, planks, and even one-leg box jumps), but I had never had to hold something heavy overhead while balancing above muddy ground in the middle of the forest, wet and freezing cold from swimming across the lake to get to the balance beam course. Ethan was able to express strength and balance while dealing with the elements and the different environment. Ethan showed me that fitness is only a part of the puzzle to longevity. It's an important part, to be sure, but not the whole of it. If we equate fitness with work we do inside the gym, we limit what fitness is and who can participate in it. The more broad and inclusive we can make fitness, the more fit we will all truly be.

Perhaps you have heard of Blue Zones. It's a term coined by Dan Buettner, a National Geographic Explorer who, building on the work of Gianni Pes and Michel Poulain, identified the five places around the world where people not only lived the longest but enjoyed a "high quality of life in their old age."[34] The five Blue Zones are Sardinia, Italy; Ikaria, Greece; Okinawa, Japan; Loma Linda, California (the Seventh Day Adventist community); and the Nicoya Peninsula, Costa Rica. The health data that comes out of these communities is impressive: less disease, lower health care costs, more happiness, greater life expectancy, and more robustness later in life. In other words, the old people are still active, healthy, and disease-free. They are cooking, gardening, socializing, walking, and enjoying life beyond their 80s and into their 90s and, for some, into their 100s.

The more I read about these places, the more I see why life is longer and more fulfilling. They live closer to one another, often with generations of family and friends, and they eat foods that are simple whole foods, seasonally prepared in delicious traditional ways. "Centenarians in all five Blue Zone areas enjoy much lower rates of chronic disease like obesity, heart disease, type 2 diabetes, and dementia. They eat a plant-slant diet of whole foods; fruits and vegetables are present at every meal, lowering inflammation and increasing immunity."[35]

I do realize I've spent the previous chapters talking about the importance of closing the intensity gap, the adaptation cycle, and real strength training. And I stand by that science. But it's only part of the picture, and we don't need gyms to live long, healthy lives. After all, there are no Core Powers in Sardinia. No CrossFits on the Nicoya Peninsula. And I doubt that Planet Fitness will arrive anytime soon in Ikaria.

One of the commonalities of the populations in Blue Zones is that they move naturally because they "live in environments that constantly nudge them into moving without thinking about it. They grow gardens and don't have mechanical conveniences for house and yard work."[36] This is called N.E.A.T. (non-exercise activity thermogenesis).

Even the hardest workout you will ever do in a group fitness class (think: crushing intervals, burpees, squats, push-ups, and lunges that leave you exhausted and torched) will only burn 13 percent of your daily calories. Now think about being active throughout the day: walking more than 10K steps, standing most of the time instead of sitting at your desk, working with your hands, or getting out for a hike after dinner instead of watching TV.[37] This—N.E.A.T.—burns up to 30 percent of daily calories, and is a way of life.[38] But before you think about replacing your interval or strength training with N.E.A.T., remember that you still need strength training to elicit a hormonal response. It's about balance. And there are some simple ways to make impactful changes to your N.E.A.T. Try and shoot for 10K steps a day or more. Take walking meetings on the phone or in person. Go for a walk after dinner, first thing in the morning, or over lunch.

Growing up, my parents were very busy. My dad was an English teacher at a public high school. In the evenings, he sold car parts at Sears. On the weekends, he worked at The Pickle Barrel, my uncle's deli in east downtown Des Moines, Iowa. (It had to have been the only Jewish delicatessen in Iowa at the time and they had the best corned beef on rye!) My mom is a first-generation immigrant from Mexico and she was a full-time high school Spanish teacher and attended school in the evenings working toward her master's degree in education. It was the '80s and the gym scene wasn't what it is today; there were no 5:00 AM boot camp classes they could hit before school started (and that wouldn't have occurred to them). Instead, we walked, we went on bike rides, and we found ways to move, together. Most nights after dinner we would go for a walk or my dad and I would play basketball in the driveway. We were usually all in bed by 10:00 PM, so we got a good night's sleep. Without knowing it, my parents were creating lifestyle habits that went a long way for them and us.

My parents are now in their mid-80s. Both are healthy and still very active. As they've aged, I've noticed that their lifestyle choices have been a significant part of what keeps them healthy. Every time I go back to Iowa for a visit, we walk everywhere; it's part of how we connect. We cook and share meals together, everyone sitting around the huge dining room table. If my brother and sister and their families are there, we number 21. It's family, so it's not always perfect, but the healthy lifestyle habits my parents modeled for us allow my siblings and I to remain connected, healthy, and happy.

Just as with fitness, lifestyle and nutrition have to be sustainable in order to have real impact. Quick fixes and the latest fads rarely work over time. Instead, making simple changes to how we live our daily lives can be the most impactful things we will do in our wellness journey. The key is learning to be a critical thinker, not just about your fitness, but about your lifestyle and nutrition, as well.

Sitting

The amount of time you spend sitting can significantly affect your health. A friend recently joked that, "sitting is the new smoking." Well, not exactly, but there is a growing body of research that demonstrates the dangers of sitting too much. A study published in the *Journal of Lifestyle Medicine* found that for each daily two-hour increment of sitting, the risk of diabetes and obesity went up 5 percent and 7 percent, respectively. The same study also revealed that greater overall sitting time is associated with muscle loss. Specifically, for each additional hour of sitting over eight hours per day, there was a 33 percent increase in muscle loss.[39] And in 2013, the World Health Organization (WHO) estimated that 3.2 million people died prematurely from a sedentary lifestyle.[40] According to Just Stand.org, you are low-risk if you sit for less than four hours daily,[41] and you are considered sedentary if you sit for six or more hours per day.[42] More than 60 percent of adults in the U.S. are considered sedentary,[43] which puts them at a 20–30 percent higher risk of all-cause mortality.[44]

Sitting too much is also a common cause of skeletal and soft tissue injury. Sitting for long periods shortens the front of the hip and causes the glutes to become inactive. This was my friend Kate's problem. This can cause hip problems and lower back problems. Sitting with poor posture can cause upper back problems and shoulder problems.

So, just stop sitting as much? Yup, that's part of the solution. But if you know you've been sitting too much and have a related injury or imbalance, you will have to address that before you can fully dive into a new training program. This means developing a practice that stretches whatever is tight and activates whatever is inactive. See the Appendix for assessments and stretches for injuries and imbalances related to sitting.

Other things to consider to reduce how much you are sitting: set up a standing desk at work and try to work standing as much as possible; instead of sitting while watching TV, use the time for foam rolling or stretching; if you must sit, try to get up every 30 minutes and walk or stand for five minutes.

Sleep

During the first five years of our marriage, Christine and I had three kids, we'd opened a boutique fitness studio, I was a full-time performance coach for a professional soccer team, and I was managing the fitness of two Olympic athletes. I was often traveling with the team or one of my athletes, and when I wasn't traveling, I would wake up at 4:00 AM to head into the studio, often not getting home until 9:00 PM. I didn't necessarily feel tired; I just kept going.

In the meantime, Christine was at home with three kids ages three and under. She was doing administrative work for the studio between changing diapers, going to the park, and (likely) plotting ways to kill me for not being around to help. As much fun as it was being a young family, we were both exhausted. What I learned later was that "tired" had become our "normal." I didn't realize it until a friend invited us to spend a relaxing week at his vacation house in Palm Springs. For the first time in over five years, we had nothing to do and no schedule to follow. We went to bed early and slept later. I actually feel like I slept for the first four days. When I woke up on day four, it seemed like the world was different, effervescent.

I was more creative, in a better mood, could see things clearly, and felt different—happier.

I tell everyone how important sleep is, so I'm embarrassed to admit that I was not taking care of myself, and my lack of sleep was affecting my mood, fitness, work, and relationships. After learning this lesson the hard way, I changed my sleep schedule and sleep habits. It wasn't as easy as just going to bed earlier and waking up later; I needed to understand what was getting in my way, and that took time and reflection. I realized I needed to let go of some of the pressures I had put on myself to build a business, satisfy clients, and travel with the team. Eventually, I was able to create more balance and restore healthy sleep. Christine appreciated this because she needed my help and I was able to spend more time at home. I would take the kids for walks, help make dinner, and Christine was able to catch a few breaks to start to restore some of her sleep, as well.

How much sleep is ideal for adults ages 40–60? Seven to nine hours, depending on activity level and what feels right. Sleep deprivation can cause impaired judgment, slow reaction times, a weak immune system, and weight gain. When you don't get enough sleep, the hormones that control hunger and fullness don't function properly and lead to overeating.

Sleep quality is also important. Sleep aids don't help with sleep quality. They put you to sleep but don't allow you to get to deep sleep and rapid eye movement (REM) sleep, where physical and emotional recovery occurs. Here are a few simple things to try if you are having trouble sleeping:

1. Create a blackout room, with no natural light from windows and no artificial light from phones, alarms, computers, etc.

2. Keep your room cool. Maintaining a temperature between 60–68 degrees helps with sleep quality. Our bodies lower their normal temperature by about two degrees Fahrenheit approximately two hours before bed. This lowering of body temperature cues the brain to release melatonin, which aids in your ability to fall asleep and stay asleep. A lower room temperature can help support the release of melatonin.

3. Get off all screens about one hour before bed. Screens give off blue light, which cues our bodies to stop producing melatonin, thus making it difficult to fall asleep.

4. Compress tissue before bed. If you have a tough time falling asleep, try using a foam roller or lacrosse ball to compress muscle and tissue right before bed. Compressing muscle and tissue, like in a deep massage, can help turn the "on switch" off.

5. Try melatonin. Melatonin is a hormone released from the brain to help with sleep, but if you are having trouble sleeping, ask your doctor about taking over-the-counter melatonin. According to the Mayo Clinic's research, it is effective in helping with all kinds of sleep disorders, including insomnia, jet lag, and delayed sleep. The Cleveland Clinic suggests starting with 1mg of melatonin before bed and increasing by 1mg as needed, not to exceed 10mg.[45]

Nutrition

Nutrition is a fraught subject for many people because we live in a society that promotes fad diets as a way to attain socially acceptable yet unrealistic—and often unhealthy—bodies. Real, sustainable nutrition is not about counting calories, measuring macros, and following fad diets. Just like fitness, real nutrition is sustainable and individualized and doesn't have to be extreme.

Nutrition Myths

Myth 1: Since I'm working out, I can eat whatever I want.
Truth: You can't out-train a poor diet.

Myth 2: I'm doing a new diet that worked for (fill in supermodel or celebrity name here) and they lost 20 lbs in 30 days, so I will, too.
Truth: We all respond differently to different diets at different times. What works for you might not work for me. What worked for me 20 years ago might not work for me today.

Myth 3: I have to lose weight quickly, so I'm doing this extreme detox/diet to lose weight in a few weeks.
Truth: Nutrition is not easy, it's not quick, and it's not effective unless it's sustainable. As we age, it's important to lean on the basics of nutrition rather than the fad diets and quick fixes.

I've seen it a million times...you think you must do something extreme to get yourself out of the hole and kickstart a new chapter in your wellness. So you go for the crazy restrictive diet or the detox that limits calories to the point where you're miserable, can't focus, can't exercise, and you end up gaining it all back anyway. Instead, if you follow the basics of nutrition, it simply becomes a sustainable way of living and eating, with no dieting required. The basics are simple: Eat minimally processed whole foods and limit sugar and alcohol intake.

Is it really that simple? Yes, actually it is.

The tricky thing is that many of us think we eat a certain way, but when we look at our food intake on paper, we realize we've actually moved far from the basics. I suggest keeping a three-day food journal, recording everything you eat and drink over three days without making changes in what you typically do. Just like fitness testing, it's a great way to see where you are right now. Once you have that information, you can move forward with a realistic nutrition plan focused on the basics. For some of you it might work better to look back two or three days and write down what you ate and drank. We have a tendency to make different decisions around food and alcohol when we know we have to record it and report it. Which actually makes journaling a great way to hold yourself accountable.

I have seen many clients begin solving problems by doing just this. Journaling and recording food and alcohol consumption. This ties into being present and active as a health consumer. For many of us, we don't think about what we eat or how much we drink, but journaling can help us think about choices. Of course, I'm old-school, something about putting pen to paper feels good. It's slower, and for this reason it also makes me think and reflect. However, there are tons of apps you can use for food journaling.

I like MyFitnessPal, which is easy to use and easy to share with a coach or friend.

Whole Foods

We're going to revisit the Blue Zones. In *The Blue Zones Secrets For Living Longer*, Dan Buettner describes the nutrition habits of each Blue Zone, highlighting the fact that people in each of these zones eat minimally processed whole foods—simple foods that taste delicious. They are eating whole grains, legumes, and green leafy vegetables. Minimally processed whole foods are denser in vitamins and minerals. They make you feel full longer, help you feel more satisfied, and are anti-inflammatory.

Tips for identifying whole foods:

1. Most whole foods are at the perimeter of the grocery store: fresh vegetables, fruit, meat, and fish are all on the outside aisles of the grocery store. Try to avoid the inside aisles as much as possible when grocery shopping.

2. If it comes in a package, read the label. If there is an ingredient you wouldn't typically have in your kitchen, think twice before buying it. I don't know about you, but I don't typically have sodium benzoate, calcium propionate, or potassium sorbate (all chemicals used to preserve processed foods) on the shelf in the pantry at home.

3. A primarily plant-based diet has been shown to increase longevity, but this doesn't mean you can't have protein. Protein is dense in minerals and vitamins. Most importantly, protein will help keep you from losing muscle. Your protein should be lean

and unprocessed, like chicken, lean cuts of beef, eggs, freshly caught fish, and other lean animal protein. For those of you who are vegetarian or vegan, beans, lentils, and even spinach can be a good source of protein.

Why are processed foods so bad?

Processed foods can force us to crave more calories, and many processed foods have an addictive quality. Our brains weren't wired to eat something crunchy, salty, creamy, and sweet all at the same time. We have a tough time putting that type of delicious-ness down. Have you ever not consciously eaten a whole pint of ice cream or finished off an entire bag of potato chips? The *British Medical Journal (BMJ)* reviewed several studies that show a strong correlation between processed food intake and coronary heart disease as well as an increased risk of cardiovascular disease. The findings were that just a 10 percent increase in processed intake daily led to a 13 percent and 12 percent increased risk of coro-nary heart disease and cardiovascular disease, respectively.[46] The Environmental Working Group reviewed a 2023 study from the *Journal of the American Medical Association (JAMA)* that links an increase in processed food intake with a 50 percent increased risk of depression in participants over the course of four years.[47]

Why are whole foods so important as we age?

As discussed earlier, as we age, we are in a hormone free fall. Our bodies are changing as we lose muscle and gain body fat. We must continue to think about how we progress with fitness to combat the decline, but we must also understand the nutrition that will support robust health, lean muscle, and high energy.

Tips for eating more whole foods:

1. Start by clearing out processed foods from your house. If it's in the house, someone is going to eat it.

2. Have seasonal fruit and other whole foods displayed. We always keep a bowl of apples sitting out in the fall, berries in the summer, etc. If it's sitting out and you can see it, it will likely be eaten.

3. Missing that snack you love? Need ideas on what to eat? There are many great resources for healthy cooking. You can recreate a more healthful version of almost anything you get in a package. I love ice cream. I make a healthier version using coconut milk sweetened with maple syrup, vanilla extract, and dark chocolate chips. Those are the only ingredients, and it's delicious and easy to make. See the Appendix for a list of my favorite websites for healthy cooking.

4. Be sure to salt your food once you are on a whole-foods diet. Your body needs sodium, which is an electrolyte. You were probably getting too much of it when you were eating more processed foods, but when you transition to whole foods, you might need to supplement. If you don't get enough sodium, you'll feel lethargic, get headaches, and feel hangry. You need around 2,000 mg daily, depending on your activity level. This is approximately 1½ teaspoons of salt.

5. If you are not one for cooking meals from scratch and prefer going out or ordering in, get used to reading labels and asking

questions. Many great healthy restaurants serve whole foods that are better than eating at a typical fast food place. Making good decisions on where you get your takeout is important. Find places that work best for you.

Sugar

Sugar is everywhere. According to the USDA, the average American eats up to 142 grams of sugar daily. That's about 34 teaspoons of sugar per day. High-sugar diets contribute to elevated blood sugar levels, insulin resistance, and leptin resistance (the hormone that tells us we are full and helps us stop eating). All of these are linked to higher body fat percentages and weight gain.[48]

The CDC recommends that no more than 10 percent of daily calories come from added sugar. That is about 50 grams for a 2,000-calorie-a-day diet.[49] In Sardinia, Italy, one of the Blue Zones, the average daily sugar consumption is less than 3 percent of daily calories. That is approximately 17 grams for a 2,000-calorie-a-day diet.[50] Sardinia has less than a 14.9 percent obesity and overweight rate,[51] versus the United States, which has a 47.3 percent obesity and overweight rate.[52]

I have seen the impact of sugar on the athletes with whom I've worked. It affects performance, injury prevention, endurance, sleep, immunity, and body composition. Sugar stimulates a physiological stressor reaction that provokes adrenal fatigue, cortisol release, and thickens the blood. This means it causes long-term fatigue, releases a stress hormone that decreases performance, and lowers the body's ability to take in oxygen. Sugar disables the immune system by compromising white blood cells, so you get sick more easily and don't recover as quickly. Sugar decreases the body's production of leptin. When insulin levels are high from too much added sugar, leptin can't do its job of signaling to us that we are full, which forces you to overeat, crave more sugar, and will eventually begin to throw off things like sleep, alertness, and decision-making ability under stress. And lastly, sugar increases oxidative stress in the body, which means you can't recover quickly or effectively.

We're not used to looking at sugar content in our products, and many products marketed toward athletes contain a lot of sugar. I always posted the following in team locker rooms to help bring awareness to athletes:

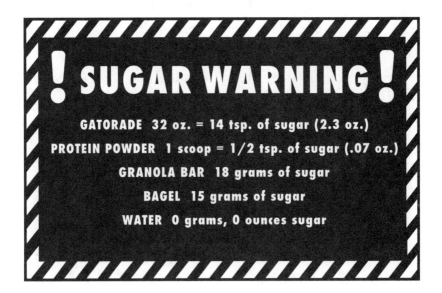

! SUGAR WARNING !

GATORADE 32 oz. = 14 tsp. of sugar (2.3 oz.)
PROTEIN POWDER 1 scoop = 1/2 tsp. of sugar (.07 oz.)
GRANOLA BAR 18 grams of sugar
BAGEL 15 grams of sugar
WATER 0 grams, 0 ounces sugar

Alcohol

As we know from looking at the Blue Zones, having one or two glasses of wine daily is common in many cultures that have a high number of centenarians, but if we isolate alcohol consumption and take out movement, nutrition, lifestyle, and socialization—the other positives in Blue Zones—the effects of alcohol look much different.

Much of our metabolism is controlled by our thyroid. Even a small amount of alcohol can cause the thyroid to be underactive. That might not be a big deal in our 20s and 30s, but as we age, our metabolism slows down anyway, so alcohol isn't helping.

Alcohol is a sleep disruptor. You may fall asleep, but you won't be able to stay asleep and get into REM sleep, where most hormones are released and abundant recovery and adaptation occur. In one study, when participants drank alcohol, they had only 8 percent of total sleep in REM. When they didn't drink, they had 25 percent of sleep in REM, which is normal.[53]

The CDC recommends no more than two drinks daily for men and one for women.[54] Of course, the U.S. sits at number 10 among the unhealthiest countries in the world, partly due to its alcohol consumption levels, which for many far exceed these recommendations.[55] In 2023, the World Health Organization came out with a statement based on years of research saying that, "No level of alcohol consumption is safe for our health."[56]

I'm not saying you can never drink alcohol. We are all affected differently by different types and doses of alcohol. I encourage you to figure out what works best for you, and notice how you feel when you do drink versus when you don't drink. I encourage my clients to reduce alcohol consumption and see if there is an effect on how they feel, sleep, and on their body composition. Often when my clients quit drinking cold turkey, it becomes a temporary change. The people who are strategic about setting realistic goals see more lasting change in their drinking habits. The strategies to decrease alcohol consumption sustainably are simple. If you are drinking three glasses of wine a night, set your limit at two. If you are drinking two, set your limit at one or schedule a dry day. Before you have your second evening drink, have two glasses of water. Use a smaller glass for alcoholic drinks. The "sober curious" movement is growing across the U.S., and with that, there are a growing number of resources that can help you be more mindful about your alcohol consumption. A quick internet search will provide many resources to help you cut back or quit drinking alcohol.

Just a little bit better

A good rule to live by with nutrition is to just make it "a little better." This actually applies to anything you are doing when it comes to your health. I've seen so many people sign on to an extreme diet or detox and then get overwhelmed by all the rules and advice they get. Many of us feel like we must commit and jump all in on whatever we try. I get it. When you realize you must lose weight or get back in shape or when something goes wrong with your health, it feels urgent and it's easy to overcommit. But this usually isn't a sustainable approach. Most of the time, the best place to start is by making things a little better. Going from not doing anything for fitness and being wholly sedentary to jumping into boot camp class seven days a week isn't a great idea. Instead, start with just going for a walk. Nutrition is similar. Going from a diet of processed, high-sugar, fast food for most meals to an all-whole-foods diet is often not sustainable. Instead, think about making small changes. Switching from a Big Mac to a Subway sandwich is a little better.

One of my buddies runs a huge real estate development business in Minneapolis. He also is the largest owner of a well-known fast-food chain. He's a busy guy who works in an environment that doesn't promote health. He gets up at 4:00 AM and goes all day, seven days a week. Most evenings are filled with client dinners or social gatherings. At first, he could sustain this lifestyle by drinking coffee all day long. Once that stopped working, he switched to soda. It took about 10 cans of high caffeine and sugar to get him through the day. After a year of this, he was pre-diabetic and had put on almost 50 lbs. When he reached out for help, he planned to drop all soda cold turkey and start working out daily. (He hadn't worked out since college 20 years earlier.) His plan lasted a week. Instead, we devised a simple plan for "just a little bit better." He had to try and get 5,000 steps in each day, and he would replace one can of soda with a can of iced tea that had less caffeine and less sugar. This was manageable, and he was able to keep it up and slowly reduce his soda intake. After six months, he was off of soda completely, he had lost 30 lbs, and his blood sugar normalized so he was no longer pre-diabetic. By re-evaluating his decisions every couple of weeks, he was able to get to a much healthier place in a sustainable way.

"A little bit better" applies to any part of your health and fitness. It's part of how you progress. As I mentioned earlier, eating whole foods is part of the basics of nutrition, but if you aren't there yet, you can make things just a little bit better by having 50 percent of your meal from whole foods or 20 percent or whatever is just a little bit better than what it was before.

The "Miracle" Diets

Most of the fad diets have something good in them. But often the good part is taken out of context or taken to the extreme. For example, the Paleo diet wasn't meant to be bacon, steak, and burgers. It was developed in the 1970s by Walter Voegtlin, who believed eating like our Paleolithic ancestors could make us healthier. This meant getting rid of all foods that come from farming, such as grains and legumes, the primary sources of carbohydrates for most people. This was meant to shift the focus from bread, pasta, and cereals to fruits and vegetables as the primary source of carbohydrates. Initially, lean protein was meant to be less than half of your daily calories. But after hitting mainstream diet culture, the Paleo diet changed. For some, it became more about anything you wanted to eat as long as it didn't have grains. Now you can pick up paleo candy bars, paleo donuts, and paleo cereal, all with the same amount of sugar and calories as their non-paleo counterparts.

Similarly, the Keto diet was developed in 1924 by Dr. Russell Wilder as a treatment for patients with epilepsy at the Mayo Clinic. The diet is very restrictive in carbohydrates, focusing on high fat and protein. The idea is that when carbohydrates are restricted or eliminated, the body switches from burning carbohydrates to burning fat. When you burn more fat as fuel for longer periods of time (weeks and months), your liver will produce ketones, which your body will use as fuel when no glucose is present. When ketones are present, your glucose levels go way down. High levels of glucose are linked to some seizures in patients with epilepsy because high levels of glucose can lead to excitability in neurons in the brain, which can, in turn, disrupt signaling in the brain and trigger a seizure. Ketones, however, have an anti-epileptic effect on the brain. It is hypothesized that this is the case because ketones are metabolically efficient and don't cause the same excitability as glucose does in the brain.[57]

In addition to potentially reducing seizure activity, the benefits of the Keto diet are weight loss, low blood sugar levels, and in some cases, an improved lipid panel, and for some athletes, enhanced performance. But the side effects of the Keto diet can include fatigue, headache, nausea, dizziness, vomiting, constipation, and low exercise tolerance. Sounds fun, doesn't it?

For most of us, fad diets aren't sustainable and, when taken to the extreme, they can be unhealthy. With that said, it's okay to experiment. It can be an excellent way for you to learn. My only caution is that you test knowing that you are doing just that, testing. Be careful not to jump into a diet that isn't sustainable for you, like the "lion diet" where you only eat meat, salt, and water. Instead, balance and getting back to the basics—whole foods and limited sugar and alcohol—is key.

80 percent rule

I just can't get behind long-term calorie counting. It's not a sustainable nutrition solution. And counting calories will never teach you to pay attention to fullness and hunger signs. I have seen thousands of people freed from counting calories when they instead shift their focus to understanding fullness and portion sizes.

There is nothing worse than being on a specific regime of limited calories and knowing that you are going to be hungry. Not only is this poor practice and sometimes unhealthy, but this can sometimes lead to weight gain due to the body holding on to fat as a way of survival. I find the people who have the most success with nutrition are the ones who take it upon themselves to be educated and understand what fullness and hunger really feel like.

The most straightforward rule in nutrition if you are trying to lose weight is to eat until you are 80 percent full. This is a foreign concept to most of us, but if you are willing to give it a try, you'll see it's easy, it feels good, and you don't have to starve yourself. Eating to 80 percent is eating until you feel satisfied, not full. You should feel like you can get up and walk away.

Start by slowing down your eating. Two hormones control hunger and fullness. When you eat too fast, the hormone that makes you feel full, leptin, doesn't signal that you are full until it's too late, and you already overate and feel stuffed. Likewise, when you eat too fast, the hormone that makes you feel hungry, ghrelin, doesn't have time to shut off. Slow it down, chew your food, set the fork down between bites. Once you know what your body feels like to be 80 percent full, you can adjust portion sizes accordingly.

Plant-Based or Carnivore?

I've worked with world-class athletes who were vegan and others who ate meat, and both have thrived. I've seen people lose weight and gain weight with both approaches. The key, again, is balance. Eat veggies and fruits and have some protein.

Once or twice a year I reset by doing an 800-gram challenge with vegetables. Nutritionist EC Synkowsky came up with the idea as a way of helping people eat more healthfully without all the diet restrictions. How it works: simply consume 800 grams of fruits and vegetables before you eat anything else.[58] Every time I do it, I walk away feeling great and resetting how I eat.

How much is 800 grams?

1 10-ounce bag of spinach = ~250 grams

1 medium cucumber = ~200 grams

1 medium tomato = ~120 grams

2 cups of fresh blueberries = ~300 grams

1 apple = ~70 grams

If you want to try the challenge, it's a great way to reset, get more veggies in your diet, and learn new ways to prepare them. The guidelines:

1. Fresh, frozen, raw, steamed, baked, and grilled all count.
2. No dried fruits, which contain too much sugar without enough nutrients.
3. Eat 800 grams or more of vegetables before you eat anything else.
4. Try it for a week. I usually end up going longer because I feel so good.
5. You might want a food scale, which you can find online for under $10.

Whenever I do this, I learn new recipes for breakfast, lunch, and dinner. And I've found that if I have just one vegetable on the table when my family sits down for a meal, it doesn't get eaten. But if I have a variety of three or four different vegetables on the table, they all end up being eaten.

Body Type

For most people, thinking about how to eat or train according to body type isn't necessary. Staying connected to the basics, being aware of why you are doing what you are doing, and progressing are great guidelines for a path forward. But if you are stuck, looking at body type is a viable option.

The older I get, the more surprised I am at how different people adapt to different diets, training methods, and lifestyle changes. I have seen two people make the same changes to nutrition, and only one person is affected. I see this most often in partners. For example, they both will limit alcohol and one will lose 10 lbs right away, while the other will see no change even though both drank the same amount and gave up the same amount. I see it happen with training, as well. In a group training for a race and following the same training program, some people lose weight, some gain weight, and some maintain the same weight. The same goes for performance; some adapt to a specific stimulus while others see no change. I'm certain some of you have experienced this when you see a friend go on a specific diet or try a specific exercise protocol, and it works amazingly well for them, but it does nothing for you. One of the ways we can start to answer the question and change the outcome is to look at body type.

After seeing how people respond to different nutrition and training styles, I realized that much of our response is based on our genetics. How our body looks naturally can indicate how our genetics might respond to different types of nutrition and training. We are all different, but looking at body type can help us refine and make the best guesses regarding training and nutrition. I'm not talking about drastic changes, but instead little tweaks to your nutrition and training to support improvements.

Not everyone fits into one of the three body types. Some of you will know right away what body type you are, and some will feel like you might be a mix of two different body types. You will still have some guidance based on your mix of body types. We can identify with body type not just through visualization, but by knowing how you respond to certain nutrition and types of training.

The three general body types are:

Ectomorph: They are lean, long, and skinny. Think Cameron Diaz in *There's Something About Mary* or Brigid Kosgei, the famous marathon runner and two-time winner of the London and Chicago Marathons and silver medalist in the 2020 Olympics.

Mesomorph: They are muscular and can easily gain and lose weight. Think Brad Pitt in *Thelma and Louise* or a track and field 100-meter sprinter.

Endomorph: They carry more body fat, are a bit more burly, and sometimes feel like they gain weight by simply looking at a cheeseburger. Think Serena Williams's 1999 Grand Slam win or a football player lineman.

ECTOMORPH	MESOMORPH	ENDOMORPH

It's important to remember when looking at body types that you can't change your genetics. You can never go from endomorph to ectomorph. No matter how much you starve yourself, it just won't happen. Learn to love your body and reach toward making it healthier. When you place the focus on health and movement, it can lower body image stress.

Each body type metabolizes proteins, carbs, and fats differently. This is why a single diet doesn't work for everyone. Take carbs, for example. Ectomorphs can typically eat more carbs without gaining much weight. Carbs not used as fuel are stored as fat, and the ectomorph is more efficient at burning carbs because they usually have a higher resting metabolic rate. Mesomorphs tend to gain more muscle when they eat more protein and lift weights. They have more fast twitch muscle, and that type of muscle can increase in size easier than slow twitch muscle, which is what a mesomorph typically has more of. Endomorphs often gain weight quickly with carbs because they have a slower metabolism and not as much lean muscle.

If you are wondering if you have more fast twitch muscle fibers or slow twitch muscle fibers, you can probably tell by what type of training you are drawn to. I am more slow twitch and loved marathons. My wife is more fast twitch and prefers short sprints. I also use an app called CNS Tap Test, which creates a place in the middle of your phone screen to tap. Simply tap your phone with your index finger as fast as you can for 10 seconds. How many taps you get will give you an idea of what type of muscle fiber you predominantly have. For example, I'll tap 50 taps in 10 seconds while my wife will tap 100 times in 10 seconds. Again, muscle fiber type and body type are not always precisely linked, but it can be helpful to have this information.

I am sure you have something in common with one or more of these body types and the descriptions of typical weight gain or loss associated with each one. That's good and useful information for you.

As you read through the prescriptions of nutrition and exercise, understand that these are not magic solutions, just general guidelines. You must be willing to jump in and make changes based on what you think you need. Try it, reassess, adjust, and continue until you are starting to see results. It won't happen overnight.

The following are my most common recommendations for body types based on longevity, health, and robustness: an ectomorph needs to gain lean muscle, a mesomorph needs to understand how to balance everything, and an endomorph generally needs to lose body fat.

Nutrition for Body Type

The ideal body fat percentage for women 40–59 is 23–33 percent, and for men of the same age it is 11–22 percent.[59] For **endomorphs,** limiting carbohydrate intake can be a good place to start, making sure the carbohydrates you are consuming are from whole food sources as much as possible.

35 percent lean protein

25 percent whole food carbohydrates

40 percent healthy fats

You don't have to measure this all out; simply know more protein and fat and less carbohydrates.

Ectomorphs probably want to find ways to gain lean muscle. A quick reminder that as we talk about aging, our language changes from a six-pack to bone density, from ripped quads to optimal hormones and lean muscle. A recent study showed a strong link between longevity and more lean muscle in arms and legs.[60] I'm not saying that a six-pack and ripped quads can't be done at your age; they can, but the focus is first on health and a big part of that for this body type is building lean muscle. This might be a good start for you to think about how to break up your macronutrients:

35 percent lean protein

45 percent whole food carbohydrates

20 percent healthy fats

Again, you don't have to count everything; make it easy with more carbs, less fat, and more protein.

For **mesomorphs**, it's easier to gain muscle and lose fat, so a more balanced approach is a good place to start. Again, you can dial this up or down based on your needs. More carbohydrates might help with performance and fewer carbohydrates might help with weight loss. Remember that lean muscle is important as we age, and protein intake is a big part of that.

30 percent lean protein

40 percent whole food carbohydrates

30 percent healthy fats

Fitness by Body Type

If you want to tailor your fitness to your body type, first make sure you are following the intensity guidelines I laid out for the adaptation cycle of stimulus and fatigue. Remember the story of my friend Mary, who ran the marathon and gained weight because her training was lacking intensity? In other words, don't confuse the number of reps, the rest, and the number of sets as the magic formula because it's not. By following the prescriptions below, you'll see change, but only if you have the correct intensity.

If you are new to intensity, new to strength training, and new to pushing yourself to the edge, this will take you some time. Be willing to experiment just a little bit at first. You'll know when you have gained confidence and feel comfortable enough to test the limits. The last five repetitions of each set of strength training should be challenging. That means that those repetitions will get sticky, they won't be smooth, you may get stalled on a few. Your heart rate should skyrocket after a set. You should be out of breath, as if you just finished a sprint. If you have never done anything like this, it will take at least six weeks for you just to get comfortable and gain motor control over what you are doing in order to challenge yourself with the load.

How do you progress? You can follow the 2 x 2 rule. If on the last two sets you can do two more repetitions than you have set out to do, then go up in weight for the next workout. It's typical to go up 3–5 lbs for the upper body and 10–20 lbs for the lower body.

The following plan is for an endomorph who wants to train for weight loss. (This plan will also work for any body type who wants to train to lose weight.)

- Interval training of 2 minutes or more with a 1:1 work-to-rest ratio. 3–5 efforts
- Weight training should consist of lighter loads with higher reps. 5+ sets of 15 or more repetitions. The last five repetitions should be challenging for each set.

ENDOMORPH
Goal: Weight loss

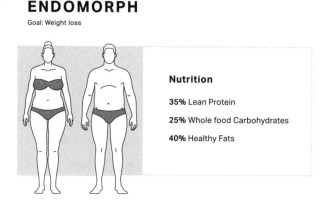

Nutrition

35% Lean Protein

25% Whole food Carbohydrates

40% Healthy Fats

TRAINING

Power   *Strength*   *Endurance*

For a mesomorph who wants a balanced training approach, look at the full spectrum of training adaptation as it applies to reps and sets. This body type can see adaptation working with high reps and endurance cardio to low reps and sprints. The key is finding the balance.

- Weight training should consist of moderate to heavy loads with mid-range repetitions. 4+ sets of 8–12 repetitions.
- Interval training of 30 seconds up to 2 minutes with a 1:2 work-to-rest ratio. 10–20 efforts.

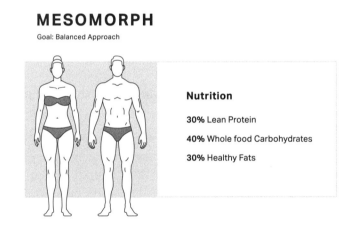

MESOMORPH
Goal: Balanced Approach

Nutrition

30% Lean Protein

40% Whole food Carbohydrates

30% Healthy Fats

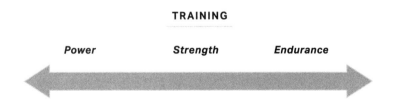

TRAINING

Power   *Strength*   *Endurance*

The following plan is for an ectomorph who wants to gain muscle.

- Weight training should consist of very heavy loads with low repetitions. 3+ sets of 1–5 repetitions.
- Interval training of 10 to 30 seconds with a 1:3 work-to-rest ratio. 25–30 efforts.

Remember that as we age, it's really hard to add bulk, but if you are so inclined, give this training style a shot and pair it with a higher protein diet.

ECTOMORPH
Goal: Gain Lean Muscle

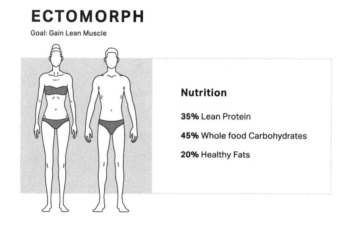

Nutrition

35% Lean Protein

45% Whole food Carbohydrates

20% Healthy Fats

TRAINING

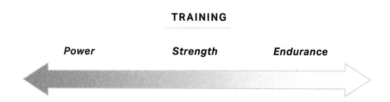

Power   *Strength*   *Endurance*

Intermittent Fasting

The chatter surrounding intermittent fasting has increased significantly in the past few years. Not surprisingly, much of the recent research around fasting and weight loss needs to be more conclusive. What we do know is that long-term studies of intermittent fasting show links to increased longevity[61] and chronic disease prevention,[62] but no link to sustainable, long-term weight loss. Given the benefits, the many options for fasting, and my propensity to experiment on myself, I decided to try a few options to see the effects.

24-Hour Weekly Fast

I started with a 24-hour fast one time per week for seven weeks.

Difficulty Level:

Very difficult at first to moderate at the end. I fasted from Wednesday after dinner to Thursday evening, my lighter training day. My first couple weeks were challenging: low energy on fasting days, moody and hungry. By the third or fourth week, it got much easier, and by the end, I could have kept doing it week after week. It seemed manageable in terms of difficulty.

The Positives:

I learned how to manage hunger. The fasting taught me that it was okay to be hungry and that I would be okay without having to eat every two to three hours.

The Negatives:

I didn't like missing meal times with my family. Sometimes, my 24 hours would fall later than our normal dinner time, and I would have to just sit at the table without eating. Family meals are big in our house, and I don't want to change that part of my lifestyle. Because my fast days were planned, I also tended to overeat before and after, and it didn't feel great to feel stuffed on Wednesday and Thursday evenings.

12-Hour Daily Fast

For my second experiment, I moved to a 12-hour fast every day of the week for eight weeks, basically from 8:00 PM after dinner to 8:00 AM the next day.

Difficulty Level:

Super easy. I never felt hungry and got into a simple habit of eating a quick snack at 8:00 AM even if I wasn't hungry. Otherwise, I felt like my training sessions would have been low energy.

The Positives:

I felt great because I never felt hungry. It was easy to manage this type of fasting and not overeating because I didn't feel like I was ever fasting.

The Negatives:

Again, lifestyle! I was missing out on early morning family breakfast on weekends. We usually wake up and make some kind of banana bread, muffins, eggs, and turkey bacon. I missed out on that.

16–18-Hour Random Fast

My third experiment was a 16–18 hour fast randomly 3–5 times per week for four weeks.

Difficulty Level:

Moderately difficult at first, but after about two weeks, I was in a routine that worked. I would sometimes feel hungry, but not the kind of hungry that all I could do was think about food.

The Positives:

This fit into my lifestyle. I had the freedom to fast after the last meal of the day, and the next day, I had a late lunch and that worked well for me. I never had to miss a family meal, and I had my weekend early family breakfasts back.

The Negatives:

Some days were tough for me, and when I first started, I tried doing Monday through Friday fasting for 16–18 hours. Toward the end of the week, I would get tired or cranky. Also, I didn't like fasting on Fridays because we celebrate Shabbat most Fridays, so I do a lot of cooking during the day, and I don't like fasting while cooking all day. Once I adjusted to 3–5 times a week, I had the freedom to pick my fasting days and make them totally random. This helped because I didn't feel like I had to stick to a schedule and it gave me more freedom.

Now, I follow something close to 3–5 times weekly for 12–18 hours. I like to let it go with where my day is taking me. Since I have learned to control hunger from the 24-hour fast, I'm okay with being hungry for a bit. I work best with doing it all randomly.

Big Picture

Fasting can be used for longevity and chronic disease prevention. Personally, I feel better fasting because it keeps me from being a late-night snacker. I sleep better not going to bed feeling full and I wake up feeling lighter and more energetic. But the jury is still out on intermittent fasting. However, I have seen intermittent fasting used very successfully as a tool to create some boundaries and guidelines for people who are trying to create better nutrition habits around things like eating later or snacking while watching TV late at night. The no-eating time creates some clarity and sets clear boundaries on exactly when you can and can't eat. But no one method works for everyone.

If you are interested, experiment with several methods to see what works best for you. Women who are over 40 may want to be more strategic about intermittent fasting. Restricting calories when training can affect energy levels and performance during training, especially when trying to build lean muscle and increase hormones. Some women who have practiced intermittent fasting have noticed an increase in metabolism and a decrease in body fat. It all depends on genetics, fitness level, health, lifestyle, etc. As always, if you experience any abnormal symptoms like depression, nausea, dizziness, or, even in some cases, body swelling, you should stop fasting and consult a doctor.

CHAPTER 8

Creating Your Fitness Plan

As you now know, when we get too dialed into one discipline of fitness we are missing out on the broader goal of wellness. Many of you are amazing yogis but you can't run a mile or do 10 burpees in a row. Likewise, some of you are strong weightlifters but lack flexibility and cardio capacity. Those of you who have the broadest reaches in fitness across the most fitness domains are the most fit. The key to not getting caught up in one discipline is to vary your training in impactful ways and to be open to learning new training disciplines as part of a bigger plan that is always progressing. The more capacity you have in varied fitness domains, the more fit, functional, strong, fast, and younger you will look. The following sample fitness plans were developed with this in mind.

All the examples in this section are from real people who have done the fitness assessments outlined in Chapter 5. They all have Fit Scores. The goal here is to give you someone with a Fit Score similar to yours so you can see what a training program looks like for someone similar to you in terms of fitness capacity. You'll see an overview of their training program and how it was adapted to meet not just their physical but emotional needs, keeping in mind the three pillars discussed in Chapter 1: awareness, connection, and progression. Each plan uses the individual's needs, experiences, and the patterns that drive engagement to assign long-term impactful programming.

You'll notice a common theme in each of these programs. First, essential data is collected in regards to what each client's needs are in terms of connecting to fitness and health. Not everyone wants to just jump in and go for it. Some people are hesitant or dealing with injuries that cause chronic pain. Some are intimidated and scared to start their journey. All of these things play a part in how we start and how we progress. The first 14–21 days of a new fitness program is a constantly moving target because you might be just learning what you are connected to, how you deal with intensity, how quickly you can recover, and what the appropriate rate of progress is. This is a time of discovery. Some of the most potent changes you will make in your program will be in the first 2–4 weeks as you learn what works for you. There is no single path for everyone.

The Programs

Program 1: Hesitant, slow restart from scratch
Michelle was 51, a full-time ninth-grade teacher, wife, and mother of two high school students.

Fitness Check-up:

FITNESS CHECK UP: MICHELLE		
TEST	**SCORE**	**POINTS**
1-mile run	14:45	0
HR push up (2 min.)	12	1
Sit to stand (1 min.)	34	2
Sit to rise	5	3
Dead hang	2 seconds	0
	TOTAL:	6

Fit Score: 6 = Beginner

About Michelle:

I learned about Michelle's relationship to health and exercise through her intake process. She had spent the previous two years counting every calorie, planning meals, and measuring every ounce of protein, carbohydrate, and fat that went into her body. She worked with a coach who monitored her nutrition and trained her in the gym. Through this very strict process, she had lost about 50 lbs. She looked great and felt great. But then the process got to be too much for her.

Prior to being on this restrictive diet, Michelle had loved cooking and loved being creative with her cooking. It brought her joy. But with this diet plan, she was limited in what she could cook. Her Sundays were her prep days; she would prepare enough chicken, rice, and vegetables for the week and weigh and measure everything so that each day was already set for breakfast, lunch, and dinner with the right portion sizes. This meant no creative cooking. Furthermore, because she was the cook in the family and the rest of her family was not on the same restrictive diet, she was preparing separate meals for them or they were ordering takeout. Soon, that became five takeout meals a week for her family.

After two years of this, she couldn't take another day. She stopped following the diet plan and ate whatever was around the house. She didn't want to think about or deal with it, and she certainly didn't want to try something else. She quickly gained all her weight back and then some. When she came to me, she was hesitant to try another new thing that she might not be able to stick with.

Michelle had always worked hard at things. She raised two kids and worked long hours as a teacher, and at different points in her life she'd had an engaging fitness practice. She wasn't a former athlete, but she liked to be challenged. She loved dancing and she loved Zumba, but she hadn't done it in years. At home, she had a kettlebell and a few other pieces of exercise equipment, such as a medicine ball, a jump rope, and a set of 10-lb dumbbells. She had previously worked with a trainer and knew how to do some things, but wasn't confident enough in her strength practice enough to do complicated movements. Plus, she recognized her limits and how deconditioned she had become. She could run, but not for more than a couple of minutes. She could push her body weight up off

the floor, and she could jump. She didn't have any restrictive injuries that she knew about. Her goals weren't specific to weight loss.
She wanted to feel better, healthier.

It was meaningful for her to feel supported and to know she
had the autonomy to speak up and have a say in how restrictive,
challenging, and in-depth the program was. After all, she was
coming from a fitness plan that didn't take her into account; it was
just about following the rules.

Michelle was so burned out from tracking everything that
she was understandably hesitant to track anything at all. For
her program, it was important to limit what she was tracking
and equally important that she understood why tracking was an
important part of her program. I let her know about the N.E.A.T.
(non-exercise activity thermogenesis) study in regard to calorie
burn, and she was interested. I decided to only ask her to track steps
on non-training days, and I didn't want to give her a minimum.
It was best to bring more awareness to where she was currently
and let her have the autonomy to decide if she wanted to reach
higher. Of course, I gave her the information on centenarians who
covered 10K and 20K steps a day because it's important for her to
know the standard.

Nutrition was a sensitive subject for Michelle after spending
the past two years feeling like her hands were tied, and someone
was watching over her, judging her. I wanted to make sure that she
had the freedom to tackle this at a pace that worked well for her.
Following the "just a little bit better" rule seemed a good place to
start. Going from five takeout meals to four in a week is "just a little
bit better." She was aware of how important it is to eat minimally

processed whole foods, but she wasn't ready to dive in deep. The question I wanted her to ask each day was whether she'd made any decisions that were just a little bit better than what she'd been doing before. That could mean going from two cookies for dessert to one or from having no water to one glass a day.

Because I knew that Michelle loved Zumba, it was easy to put this into her week so she felt that connection. She rated her Zumba session a 4 out of 5 on the Rating of Perceived Exertion (RPE) scale. The RPE scale is 1–5, with 1 being the lowest to 5 being the highest rate of perceived exertion.

Taking into consideration what made Michelle feel connected, her awareness of her current health situation, and where she wanted to go, this is what her first week of training looked like:

DAY	TRAINING TYPE
Monday	HIIT
Tuesday	Steps (N.E.A.T.)
Wednesday	Zumba
Thursday	Strength
Friday	Steps (N.E.A.T.)
Saturday	Sprint Intervals
Sunday	Steps (N.E.A.T.)

Here is an example of her first High Intensity Interval Training (HIIT) session. Note that she rated everything on a scale showing how she perceived exertion. This helped me gauge progression and whether or not to turn up or down the intensity.

WORKOUT 1	
3 Rounds of:	**Rating of Perceived Exertion (RPE): 1-5**
Run 2 minutes	*4*
Rest 2 minutes	
20 air squats	*3.5*
5 hand release pushups	*4*
10 bent knee leg raises	*5*
Rest 1 minute	

Her strength sessions were built around the equipment that she had at home and what her fitness check-up tests showed for her capacity in upper and lower body strength. As you look through the exercises, know that Michelle had access to videos from my website and YouTube channel for each activity so she understood how to move safely and correctly.

ACTIVITY	SETS	REPS	LOAD	RPE FOR EACH ACTIVITY	RPE OVERALL
Floor dumbbell chest press	4	10–15	10 lb	*4.5*	*4.5*
Bent knee renegade row	4	8–10 per side	10 lb	*5*	
Kettlebell front squat	4	10–15	15 lb	*4*	
Lunge step	4	10 total	body weight	*4*	

Michelle's sprint sessions were a way to encourage her to run faster than her mile pace. It's important to work on range when it comes to cardio capacity. Endurance or aerobic capacity is how we burn most of our fat, but it's also good to be able to express the ability to work at higher levels of intensity for shorter periods, which is more anaerobic and uses glucose as a fuel as opposed to fat. Unused carbs, which turn into glucose, get stored as fat, so having the ability to burn glucose in short, aggressive efforts is important. As you can see in the example below, she has enough information to make sure that the intensity was where it should be for this type of an activity.

DATE	ACTIVITY	SETS	REPS	DISTANCE	REST / CORE	NOTES	RPE
	Sprint (track or field)	5	1	200 meters/ .12 miles	Up to 6 minutes after each effort Core work: -30" plank -15" side plank / side -10 teasers	*Try to get each effort in under 1'22". This should leave you very out of breath!*	*4.5*

I didn't want Michelle to burn out, so I suggested training every other day except for the Zumba and strength day, which came back to back. I encouraged Michelle to use the rating system you saw earlier in the book to help her think about how she was feeling (1–5 with 5 being very sore). And, what is her desire to train today (1–5, with 5 being very willing to train)? This allowed us to see if Michelle was getting enough recovery between sessions or if she had to change the schedule or adjust the intensity. I wanted days off to have higher fatigue and soreness scores, and lower willingness to train. I wanted mornings of training days to have lower fatigue and soreness with higher readiness to train scores.

Progression wasn't easy. The program was pretty close to functional from the beginning and only a few changes were needed in things like loads, number of reps, and recovery time. The hard part was getting Michelle to progress. For the first three weeks, she wanted to keep doing the same workouts and following the same schedule. This was understandable, as she was building confidence with her re-entry into fitness and was hesitant to take on more than she could handle. Remember that your program is about you, and taking into consideration all factors that apply to your progression is important.

Taking a step back, it was important for Michelle to see that even though she wasn't yet following a progression in her program, she was still getting stronger and more fit. She could feel it. It wasn't hurting her to stay here until she felt ready. Finally, in week four, she wanted to know what a progression would look like. Because she was just getting her confidence back and creating healthy new habits around movement, lifestyle, and wellness, I knew it was essential to make her progression slow, steady, and something that was challenging for her, but attainable. Michelle's progression was gradual. Instead of running 5 sprints, she had a range of 5–7 sprints. This gave her the autonomy to move forward when she felt ready. Eventually, she just did it. She felt safe and confident enough to go from 6 to 7 sprints. As I gave her more challenging options, she slowly took on those challenges. Once she was more confident, she moved to Phase 2 of her program, which was a totally new program built off of the new fitness check-up results she had.

Michelle chose not to track her weight. She used the fitness check-up to track her progress. She also knew that a faster mile or more squats meant more lean muscles and less fat. Over the course of three months, Michelle followed a progressive program that took who she was into consideration. Here are her three-month fitness check-up results:

FITNESS CHECK-UP:	RESULTS	POINTS	RESULTS	POINTS
ACTIVITY	OLD	OLD	NEW	NEW
1-mile run	14:45	0	11:15	1
HR push up	12	1	20	3
Sit to stand	34	2	48	4
Sit to rise	5	3	8	4
Dead hang	2 seconds	0	18 seconds	1

Old Fit Score: 6 = Beginner   New Fit Score: 13 = Novice

Michelle was happy. She had come a long way in three months. What was important to her was to feel better and she did. She was a different person—confident and happier. She had more energy and she felt more alive. She didn't have a specific goal for the next phase of her training, but she was curious about how to improve her Fit Score. She was connected to what it meant for her to see the markers increase because she was able to understand that the better her Fit Score, the healthier she felt. Most importantly, she understood that it was the work she put toward trying to improve her Fit Score that was important.

Program 2: "Been there, done that." But have you really?

Chris was a 53-year-old male and a business consultant.

Fitness Check-up:

FITNESS CHECK UP: CHRIS		
TEST	**SCORE**	**POINTS**
1-mile run	12:34	0
HR push up (2 min.)	29	2
Sit to stand (1 min.)	47	3
Sit to rise	8	4
Dead hang	55 seconds	2
	TOTAL:	11

Fit Score: 11 = Novice

About Chris:

Chris came to me with a history of trying a lot of different things for fitness. He'd worked with trainers and tried different work-outs. He was athletic and active, had a Peloton, went for runs a few times a week, and was a former high school sprinter. What was eye-opening for Chris was the fitness check-up. Based on his current activity levels, he expected his Fit Score to be more advanced. It was an a-ha moment for him. He wasn't getting as much out of his fitness as he thought he was.

The big challenge for Chris wasn't helping him get to the gym and be consistent. He was used to that and already had a movement practice that he managed on his own. Chris's challenge was to create sustainability by ensuring he was training for the right reasons. At first, when things got challenging, he wanted constant reminders about why he was there. He felt motivated by things like, "Remind why I'm here…I want to lose 10 lbs." External factors drove Chris. I knew that type of motivation wouldn't last long. That's not how effective and sustainable fitness works. I knew that in order for Chris to see lasting and sustainable fitness, he would have to connect on a deeper level with what he was doing. Instead of "I'm here because I want to lose 10 lbs," he would have to find a way to shift his thinking to: "I can't wait to figure this out and get better at my 1-mile time" or "I love getting stronger because I feel more confident the stronger I get." It takes time to make this kind of shift. We are bombarded with images of abs and 30-day restrictive challenges that promise weight loss and lean bodies. To connect and have a lasting impact, Chris would have to go deeper than seeing a change in the way he looked.

As you look through Chris's program, you'll notice that, like everyone else, Chris had a lot of changes and adjustments in his first three weeks of training. Fine-tuning the right intensity level, time for recovery, and what he liked and disliked all played a role in making adjustments. At first, there was a big gap between the intended stimulus and what Chris thought he was doing. Chris's step test in the chart on the following page illustrates this intensity gap. A step test is designed to get you as close to the maximum intensity as possible. In this case we used calories and heart rate to measure intensity along with his rating of perceived exertion (RPE). In addition to identifying intensity gaps, the step test captures predicted max heart rate, which is helpful with program design.

In the step test, you increase the intensity at every predetermined time interval. Chris used the Airdyne bike, which is a stationary bike in which both arms and legs are used to generate power. Chris started slow for 1 minute, rested for 30 seconds, and then the next minute, he had to go a little faster. At every interval, Chris had to add just one calorie as a measure, and he did this until he couldn't do it again. Here is what it looked like:

STEP TEST: AIRDYNE BIKE			
TIME	CALORIES	RPE	HEART RATE
1 minute	4	1	120
2 minute	5	2	145
3 minute	6	3	157
4 minute	7	3	160
5 minute	8	3	167
6 minute	9	3	172
7 minute	10	3.5	179
8 minute	11	4	177
9 minute	12	4.5	184
10 minute	13	5	185

When we got to the end of the stress test, Chris rated his RPE at a 5 on a scale of 1 to 5. But it was clear to me that he had more in him. My goal wasn't to push Chris to his tipping point; my goal was to teach Chris how to close that intensity gap between what he thought he was capable of and what he was *really* capable of. When Chris stopped after reaching 13 calories, with his perceived exertion at a 5—basically saying he couldn't do any more—he was still able to speak in complete sentences, he wasn't sweating, and he appeared to recover within 30 seconds of stopping. I had given Chris the subjective information of what a 5 on the perceived exertion scale looked like: completely out of breath, can't talk, heart pounding, and sweat dripping. Chris was certain he was there, but in reality, he was far from it.

Part of Chris's program design included three days of cardio. I wanted to help him build a better cardio base in order to perform better on the mile. His low score put him at higher risk of cardiovascular disease and diabetes. So, I designed a cardio training day that was called "threshold," which is the place between aerobic and anaerobic in which the body is producing lactic acid at the same time that it is able to clear it. It's performed at about 80–90 percent of max heart rate and can oftentimes feel like you are on the verge of death. I know, it sounds fun, doesn't it?

In a well-trained athlete, it's sustainable for about 20 minutes. I wanted to start Chris with just four minutes in this zone. Of course, I knew his max heart rate we were using from the step test was low, so calculating 80–90 percent of his max heart rate wouldn't really work, but I had a plan to help Chris understand his intensity gap. According to his step test max heart rate, his threshold zone was 148–166 beats per minute. All you have to do is look at the chart on the previous page and see that he rated this heart rate in this zone a 2 or 3 out of 5 on the RPE (rating of perceived exertion scale), which is not exactly an on-the-verge-of-death type rating.

When we started the threshold session, I had Chris get his heart rate to 166 and told him this was the zone he was supposed to be in and I gave him the subjective cues as to how he should feel. He agreed that it didn't feel challenging at all; it actually felt easy. We tried adding 10 beats to his goal and once he got his heart rate to 177, we would re-assess. At 177, Chris was certain that he was at the threshold. I observed that he was still able to talk in complete sentences and was barely sweating. I asked Chris to cover his watch, so he couldn't see his heart rate, and asked him to continue to work for four more minutes trying to get his heart rate to 180. I told him we could just increase his speed each minute until the four minutes were up. When Chris got to the end of the four minutes his heart rate was 182, and he was just starting to show signs of being in threshold by being out of breath, sweating, and having to focus closely on making sure he maintained speed.

After Chris experienced the gap, he understood how far he was from the intensity markers that he needed in order to see change. We adjusted the threshold program based on his new heart rate, as you can see in the chart on the next page. Note that his heart rate zone is called zone 4. This is the threshold zone. Also notice that week over week, it gets harder by adding another interval. Week 3, which is not included in the chart, was a recovery week, taking into consideration the cycle of adaptation.

I will also note here how important it is to find ways to continue to assess yourself after your program starts. The movement assessments, the step test, and all the information you gather to begin a program is great. But where the rubber meets the road is when you actually start training. It's usually during a tough training session that you can see imbalances, weaknesses, or areas that need improving show up. This is exactly how we found the right heart rate zone for Chris. And this is why most programs you see in this chapter go through a phase in the first 2–4 weeks where things change and adjust. This is to accommodate new findings that come up in an authentic environment under intensity.

WEEK 1			
ACTIVITY	LOAD	VOLUME	RPE
Cardio	HR 184–186 ~~HR 166–170~~	4 minutes in zone: 4 minutes rest x 2	4.5

WEEK 2			
ACTIVITY	LOAD	VOLUME	RPE
Cardio	HR 184–186 ~~HR 166–170~~	4 minutes in zone: 4 minutes rest x 3	5

WEEK 3			
ACTIVITY	LOAD	VOLUME	RPE
Cardio	HR 184–186 ~~HR 166–170~~	4 minutes in zone: 4 minutes rest x 1	2

WEEK 4			
ACTIVITY	LOAD	VOLUME	RPE
Cardio	HR 184–186 ~~HR 166–170~~	4 minutes in zone: 4 minutes rest x 4	4.5

FITNESS CHECK-UP:	RESULTS	POINTS	RESULTS	POINTS
ACTIVITY	OLD	OLD	NEW	NEW
1-mile run	12:34	0	9:00	2
HR push up	29	2	35	4
Sit to stand	47	3	58	4
Sit to rise	8	4	9	5
Dead hang	55 seconds	2	100 seconds	4

Old Fit Score: 11 = Novice   **New Fit Score: 19 = Advanced**

It took time and a lot of reframing, but eventually Chris was really able to connect to his fitness practice and looked forward to training and enjoying the challenges in his program not just to see weight loss, but because he felt good when he could accomplish something. This created sustainability and a desire to progress for himself.

As the next few months went by, Chris was able to close the intensity gap and he began to understand how to progress his training. He really began to understand the idea of chasing fitness and he embraced working hard and understood when to rest. I introduced Chris to a group of three other men who came to the gym at the same time he did. They all had different goals and separate programs. The four of them connected, laughed, and worked hard. It was this community and camaraderie that really connected Chris to his training. He showed up to train but he also enjoyed being with his buddies. The culture they created was fun but focused. It was different than just showing up to the gym to see your friends. They were aware, they chased fitness, and they all adapted. Eventually, Chris's need to be reminded of doing hard things to lose 10 lbs faded as he became more connected to his friends in the gym and the culture they created around wellness. Chris lost more than 10 lbs and got into the best shape of his life, but more importantly, he found a connection in his movement practice.

Program 3: Never done anything like this before

Annie is a 48-year-old female who had never been in a gym before. She has disabilities that have kept her from doing strength training in the past.

Fitness Check-up:

FITNESS CHECK-UP: ANNIE		
TEST	**SCORE**	**POINTS**
1-mile run	07:25	4
HR push up (2 min.)	15	1
Sit to stand (1 min.)	45	3
Sit to rise	10	5
Dead hang	20 sec.	1
	TOTAL:	14

Fit Score: 14 = Novice

About Annie:

Annie had never worked out in a gym before because she didn't feel comfortable due to vision and balance restrictions she'd had since childhood. But Annie wanted to be a more competitive runner. She loved to run and was a good runner, as you can see from her 1-mile time trial. She also was concerned about her bone density and overall strength.

Annie's disability made it difficult for her to create stability when she moved. She was always off-balance, and when she ran, her arms and legs would flail around. So we started by creating stability in simple positions like planks and squat holds—isometric exercises that I mentioned in Chapter 3. This helped Annie understand what tension and stability in her system felt like.

Over a few months, Annie learned how to find stability and feel strong in positions. The slower her strength movements, the more she could stay connected to them and own the different positions each strength movement expressed. Her push-ups were slow, but she used her hands to connect with the floor to create stability, and she understood how to turn her core on to protect her spine.

What helped Annie enjoy and connect with her practice was figuring out how to intersperse running intervals into her workouts. As you can see in her program below, Annie would run an interval anywhere from 1–4 minutes aggressively, to the point that she was out of breath, and then while she was out of breath and tired, I would challenge her to own the positions that seemed simple but were hard to do while she was tired and out of breath. It looked like "run hard and then do 1 minute plank in a stable position" or "sprint aggressively and then do 10 stable, strong squats."

WORKOUT 1			
ACTIVITY	INTENSITY	REST	NUMBER OF ROUNDS
Run 2 minutes	10 miles per hour	None	5
Plank 1 minute	Hold in stable position	2 minutes	5
WORKOUT 2			
ACTIVITY	INTENSITY	REST	NUMBER OF ROUNDS
Run 90 seconds	10.5 miles per hour	None	5
Squat x 10	Hold bottom of each squat for 5 seconds	2 minutes	5
WORKOUT 3			
ACTIVITY	INTENSITY	REST	NUMBER OF ROUNDS
Run 1 minute	11 miles per hour	None	7
Push-up x 10	Hold bottom of each push-up for 5 seconds	1 minute	7

After about three months of this type of training, Annie was ready to start to use barbells, dumbbells, kettlebells, and medicine balls. She now understood how to create stability as she moved through certain positions. This stability gave her the strength she needed to not only move better and more safely, but created the foundation for her to progress in her strength practice so she could start to do things like back squats, deadlifts, and overhead presses. Not only did Annie get stronger as she added more strength training, her bone density improved, and she also became a stronger runner because she could translate her strength into her running ability. She no longer flailed as she ran. She was efficient and stable.

FITNESS CHECK-UP:	RESULTS	POINTS	RESULTS	POINTS
ACTIVITY	OLD	OLD	NEW	NEW
1-mile run	7:25	4	6:15	5
HR push up	15	1	22	2
Sit to stand	45	3	58	4
Sit to rise	10	5	10	5
Dead hang	20 seconds	1	60 seconds	4

Old Fit Score: 14 = Novice   **New Fit Score: 20 = Advanced**

Program 4: Former pro athlete worried about getting injured
Nate is a 45-year-old male, high-level executive.

Fitness Check-up:

FITNESS CHECK UP: NATE		
TEST	SCORE	POINTS
1-mile run	07:02	3
HR push up (2 min.)	38	3
Sit to stand (1 min.)	50	3
Sit to rise	10	5
Dead hang	125 sec.	5
	TOTAL:	19

Fit Score: 19 = Advanced

About Nate:

Nate is a former professional soccer player. After he retired from playing soccer overseas, he jumped right into marriage, kids, and a full-time career that had him traveling the world. Nate and I originally met when I was a performance coach for a professional soccer team and he was head of sales for a company that sold GPS tracking systems for athletes. He knew a lot about the science of sport and we connected right away. He was busy, but exercise was still a priority for him. He worked out at home 6–7 days a week: running, burpees, push-ups, lunges, squats. Sometimes, he would follow a fitness app or find something online that looked interesting. But when he turned 45, he realized that he was not as fit as he wanted to be; he was concerned about longevity and robustness. He had been in his own exercise world for a long time, and while it was convenient, he realized his body wasn't changing, and he wasn't getting stronger. But he'd had a lot of injuries as a pro athlete, and he was hesitant about stepping outside his routine to make changes.

Nate told me how important it was to be fit and healthy. He was starting to think about aging and wanted to be healthy and active as he got older. Nate knew that he was missing some important aspects of fitness, lifestyle, and nutrition, but he didn't know exactly what was right for him. He loved his bodyweight workouts, and he was open to change but very hesitant to start because he was afraid of getting injured trying something new. He also loved mountain biking. He lived in the mountains and loved being outside on challenging terrain, biking hard.

You can see from Nate's Fit Score that he was advanced in his fitness, but he was about to enter the world of strength training using dumbbells, barbells, and kettlebells. As discussed in Chapter 4, it can take up to two years for someone who has never lifted weights to develop a solid, progressive strength practice. And Nate had several injuries that were still restrictive for him. Through the simple movement and balance assessments discussed earlier, it was clear that Nate had some imbalances. One leg was stronger than the other. Nate did a lot of sitting for work and he had very little proprioception and awareness of the way his back and spine moved when he wasn't looking in a mirror. We needed a blended approach to address his imbalances, tightness, and improve strength.

Nate felt most comfortable with a slow rate of progression. His goal wasn't to get stronger immediately; it was to build some confidence and competency. Once he felt more balanced and could perform some of the assessments more effectively, he got over the initial hump of hesitancy to push his body, and he found a great rhythm that worked for his training and his progression.

The chart on the next page lists the series of exercises that Nate did before he trained each day. Since he only had an hour in his day for training, his corrective, mobility, balance, and stability activities started off by taking up about 50 percent of his training time, and then the other 50 percent was actual workout time, but as he progressed, his blended time shifted and he spent 20 percent of his time working on correctives, mobility, balance, and stability drills and 80 percent of his time training. The point of seeing the chart below is so you can see how much detail was spent on making sure he was well-balanced and fixing movement patterns before he began complex heavy movements. There was quite a bit of relearning how to move and a lot of detail in each exercise.

Since Nate lived in a different state, much of our work was done on Zoom so I could see him move. Sometimes he would just send me a video of him performing his activities and I would help him identify areas to watch for improvement. This interaction was important for Nate, as part of what he needed was a very solid foundation of movement mechanics and a deeper knowledge base of what movement errors to watch for to avoid injury. Eventually, he had enough knowledge and awareness that he knew when he was doing something wrong and he could correct it on his own.

WARM UP & CORRECTIVES

ACTIVITY	VOLUME	LOAD	DETAILS
Good morning forward folds	4 x 5	Body weight	Pay attention to the position of your spine. Keep the lower back arched
PNF hamstring stretch	2' per side	Heavy band	Contract and relax every 30 seconds
Shin to wall	2' per side	Body weight	Contract trail leg glute
Side lying glute activateion	4 x 10 per side	Body weight	Hip and shoulder alignment
Shoulder compression using band distraction and heavy kettlebell	2' per side	KB	Upper arm pressed to back of shoulder
Single leg balance with a lateral jump and hold	4 x 10	Body weight	Keep arch of foot open in landing
Shoulder tap plank in narrow stance	4 x 30"	Body weight	No hip swivel

Nate is three months into his program and he's made some good progress. He is thoughtful about how he moves forward and knows when he is ready. Nate still does his mountain bike rides, but he is learning how to do strength training. He is injury free and getting stronger and more confident. He has learned how to use a barbell and he is doing back squats and deadlifts to increase strength. His job has picked up again, so he doesn't have as much time to dedicate to going to the gym each day, but instead of just stopping altogether, we have developed ways to work around his busy schedule that allow him to still pursue strength training. His training sessions are condensed from doing four or five different activities that might take an hour to just doing one or two activities that allow him to get it done within 30 minutes. The ability to scale up and down as his job allows is important to him. Nate is doing great and even with his busy schedule he is still progressing.

FITNESS CHECK UP:	RESULTS	POINTS	RESULTS	POINTS
ACTIVITY	OLD	OLD	NEW	NEW
1-mile run	7:02	3	6:10	4
HR push up	38	3	45	4
Sit to stand	50	3	65	4
Sit to rise	10	5	10	5
Dead hang	125 seconds	5	121 seconds	5

Old Fit Score: 19 = Advanced   New Fit Score: 22 = Advanced

CHAPTER 9

Workout Design Overview

You've done your fitness check-up, you've read through the fitness plan examples, and based on those you have a sense of where you are and what kind of plan might be appropriate for you, but you might still feel hesitant. The following will give you an idea of how to structure a workout week.

First, always warm-up! This is critical as we age. Before you get into the bulk of any training session your body should feel warm and you should be sweating. The following is a three-part warm-up that will get you ready to train.

4-Minute General Check-in and Warm-up (Check in with yourself and see how you feel.)
- Pre-training scale of soreness/fatigue and desire to train.
- Heart rate warm-up.
- Pick any two mobility activities for 2 minutes in total.

6–8 Minute Correctives (Work on weaknesses and imbalances.)
- Use this time to work on mobility issues and imbalances. (You can choose from the movement assessments and quick fixes in Chapter 3 and the Appendix or other correctives you know work for you.)
- Pick from a list of balance, single-sided, and corrective activities you need.

6–8 Minute Dynamic Warm-up (Get all the way warmed up and practice the movements you will be using for the workout.)

- Three to four minutes of cardio building from slow to fast (relaxed to focused).
- Take the activities that you will be doing and practice them.
- Strength activities can be done without load or with light load.
- Move from slow and connected to fast and aggressive.

How to set up your training week to get the most out of each day:
As you saw in the fitness plan examples, what you do for a workout each day matters and should always take into consideration the adaptation cycle. This sample training week is based on Sunday being a rest day.

Monday: Day 1

Heavy compound lift (back squat, deadlift, front squat, overhead push press)

The first training day after a rest day should show the greatest readiness and least fatigue and soreness, so this should be the training session that puts the most demand on your central nervous system. This means that the majority of your training should be strength training on this day. Note that the loading and resting parameters are different depending on whether you are working on power, strength, or endurance. Your goals, readiness to train, body type, and Fit Score will help determine your focus.

Strength Training for Power = 1–5 reps for 3–5 sets. The load should be 100 percent to 87 percent of what you can do for 1 repetition. It's okay to estimate the load as long as you follow the 2 x 2 rule discussed previously. If you can do 2 or more reps than are prescribed in the last 2 sets, you should go up in weight (3–5 lbs for upper body and 5–10 lbs for lower body) for your next training session. It may take a few weeks, but eventually you will get to the right load. Rest as needed, which should be 2+ minutes between each set. This type of strength training is not to be rushed; it is very focused, stressful, and demanding on the nervous system, and will require a year or more of experience to handle these heavy loads.

Strength Training for Strength = 5–15 reps for 5–7 sets. The load should be 87 percent to 65 percent of what you could do for 1 repetition. Same 2 x 2 rule applies here. This type of strength training has been shown to elicit the greatest amount of hormonal stimulation. A study in the National Library of Medicine, "Effects of Recovery on Acute Testosterone and Cortizol Equated to Total Body Strength Protocols," showed 8–12 reps performed at 70–80 percent of the estimated one repetition max with 1–2 minutes of rest between sets had a greater increase in anabolic hormones compared to more power and endurance sets. The key in the study was the limited rest and the use of larger muscle groups.[63]

Strength Training for Endurance = 15 or more reps for 6–8 sets. The load should be 65 percent or less of what you could do for one repetition. Same 2 x 2 rule applies here. This type of training is great for beginning strength training because the loads are manageable and you get to do a lot of repetitions, which gives you more practice.

Tuesday: Day 2

Aggressive interval training

On the second day of training you still may feel ready to train, but the central nervous system should be taxed after your heavy strength training day. Since it is still early in the week, it might be a good idea to take advantage of your readiness by doing an aggressive interval session on this day. Of course, pay attention to your readiness, as some of you who do not yet have the capacity to handle back-to-back aggressive training days may need a recovery day before another taxing session.

The duration of the interval needs to match up with a certain amount of volume and recovery. It doesn't work to haphazardly throw different time domains out there with a guess at volume (example: 1 minute work and 30 seconds rest for 5 efforts). The specifics have to be part of the prescribed workout. The beauty is that you can do this anywhere, using anything: on a bike, on the running trail, or in any gym. Here is what we know are the best combinations of time to work, time to rest, and number of efforts associated with each.

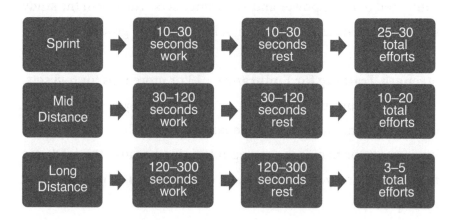

Note that your intervals have to be 95 percent to 100 percent effort! Remember that your subjective response should look and feel like this: hands on legs, heart pounding, sweating, out of breath, and feeling very, very challenged!

Wednesday: Day 3

Corrective activities and/or light training day at 60 percent intensity

Most people need to bring it down a notch after a heavy lift and aggressive intervals. If that's the case for you based on your readiness to train scores, this is a great day to focus on corrective activities. Use some of the single-sided strength activities and some of the balance activities in the Appendix. Again, if your willingness to train and soreness/fatigue is telling you to take a day off, do it here or maybe just do everything at about 60 percent of your max intensity. This could be a good day to do a light run or some easy cardio at that 60 percent intensity, or work on your yoga or Pilates practice.

Thursday: Day 4

Specific smaller muscle group strength training

Depending on how you are feeling today, it might be a good day to add another strength day into your schedule. I like to take all the big lifts and do them on Monday, but Day 4 could be a strength workout focused on smaller muscle groups, such as biceps, triceps, and core work.

Friday: Day 5

Mixed element challenge

I like Day 5! You're at the end of the week. You should be fatigued and sore, but your willingness to train should be okay. This could be another interval day, working with a different time domain, but what I like to do is a mixed element session (see the advanced fitness testing in the Appendix for ideas). I like to keep the loads light or just use body weight on Day 5 because you are already sore and fatigued, but you can still create intensity around mixing push-ups, squats, and cardio intervals. I love creating a competition on this day. Setting a goal to try and complete a certain amount of work in a specific time can drive engagement.

Sample competition

Try and complete as many rounds of the following work until you fail. Work every minute at the top of the minute as you alternate through each element:

Minute 1: 10 burpees

Minute 2: 20 air squats

Minute 3: Cardio measurable here (for example: row 10 calories, run 50 yards, bike at 150 watts)

Minute 4: Rest

Each round, increase the intensity by 1–2 burpees, 2–4 air squats, 1–2 calories, 10 yards, or 25 watts.

You can take this example or the challenges in the Appendix and scale them to fit your personal needs, like my mom does, walking up a steep hill to get out of breath. You pick what is your best starting point so that you can successfully complete at least three rounds, but no more than seven rounds.

Saturday and Sunday: Days 6 and 7
Light activity and recovery

After a week of training like this, or similar to this, it's a good idea to allow the body to recover as much as possible. Remember, Monday (or Day 1) is going to be your biggest stimulus of the week, and part of what makes that possible is your readiness and ability to be prepared to reach high on that day. On your recovery days, focus on good sleep, N.E.A.T., and clean, nourishing nutrition.

Conclusion

Remember, always, that your fitness journey is about you. It's about you owning your health and wellness. In order to do that you need to understand what works for you. The goal of sharing parts of these plans with you is to show you that fitness isn't a mystery, there isn't some secret special workout that is going to make it easier, faster, less challenging, or more effective. There is value in all movement practices, from yoga to weightlifting.

In the examples I provided, notice that each program is based on the right place to start. Looking at some of the movement assessments and seeing your Fit Score will help you decide where you need to begin. Once you know where you are on the scale of beginner to elite and as you address movement issues, injuries, or chronic pain, you can use the examples I shared as guides. That might mean taking aspects from several different plans. In the Appendix, I also outline how to design a workout and how to set up your training week to get the most of each training day, which might be helpful as you put together your progressive fitness plan.

You now understand how important it is to not just *do* fitness, but to think and feel your way through fitness. Awareness, knowing what connects you to movement, understanding why you feel a certain way about exercise, and making sure that you have balanced the cycle of adaptation with who you are and how you progress, will help you understand how to set up your program.

At the very basic level, be sure you love and are passionate about what you are doing; make sure you are following the stimulus, fatigue, recovery, and adaptation aspects of change; and make sure you have progression, that you aren't just doing the same thing week after week. You'll notice that each person in the examples had a different plan, but what they had in common were measurables, things that helped them understand and drive progression. All of their plans included strength training, and they all had some sort of higher intensity training day where they would get out of breath. How often? How much?

Those are the right questions. And I've already given you the answers. How often and how much depends on when you are ready for the next high-intensity dose of stimulus. You can measure this through the heart rate warm-up and/or by asking yourself some simple readiness questions. Am I sore? Do I have a high desire to train? Already, you are doing more than most people; you are actively participating in your fitness and wellness and thinking and feeling your way through it.

This book doesn't end here. The content is designed as a reference for you to return to again and again on your fitness journey.

When you get stuck, when you have questions, or when you want to progress, this book can be your guide. When you are uncertain of what is real, and what is healthy for you in a long-term sustainable way, use these pages as your guide. When things stop working for you, when you get frustrated, come back to these chapters to help you understand how to move forward.

Owning your fitness means you have to figure out your own path forward, based on where you are and what you need. But you now have the knowledge you need to thrive in your movement practice into the future. You've got this!

Appendix

APPENDIX A

Single-Sided Balance and Stability Exercises

As discussed in Chapter 3, single-sided exercises can help eliminate imbalances and keep you safe from future injury. The following are simple single-sided activities for the **lower body**:

1. **Single-Leg Squats:** Choose a surface that you can squat down to and touch under control. Use some form of support to help on the weaker side. You could hold onto a railing or use a resistance band tied to a stable object like a doorknob to help you lower yourself to the squat surface under control. As you get stronger on the weaker side, you'll need less and less support.

2. **Step-ups:** I like doing these as repeat reps. For example, if you are going to do 5 reps on each side, you keep one foot on the step-up surface for all 5 reps and then switch feet. On the weaker side, you may need to use your hands to push off your leg to help you get up, and that's okay as you start. You'll eventually get stronger and need less help.

3. **Lunges:** The lunge position is with your feet staggered. Your lead foot will be in front and make sure your toes point forward, your heel and big toe are down, and the arch of your foot is open. In the lead foot, keep the shin perpendicular to the floor. In the trail leg, which is behind you, your toe will be down and the heel straight up and down. Whichever leg is in front will be doing more of the work. The back leg is more of a support leg. Make sure that both sides have the same range of motion. Again, you can use your hands on your thighs to help support the weaker side until you gain strength. Lunges can be done by either moving up and down keeping feet in place, alternating by stepping forward or backward and then returning to starting position, or by walking/traveling forward or backward. They can also be done isometrically, holding a low position.

These are simple activities that, when you become comfortable, you can load by holding dumbbells, kettlebells, or barbells. Or you can do them unloaded as part of your warm-up. Another way to get some single-sided work into your workout is to do whatever you were doing but balance on one leg while doing it. TRX pull-ups on one leg, overhead press on one leg, deadlift on one leg, etc. You can be creative with implementing these activities and others that you might already be practicing, just try to do some of these single-legged activities at least one day per week.

The following are simple single-sided activities for the **upper body**:

1. **One-Arm Overhead Press:** An overhead press is performed standing with feet under hips. Whatever you are going to press overhead will be in front of your body under your chin with your forearm perpendicular to the ground. Make sure the glutes are on and your body is tight. As with a two-armed overhead press, you want to make sure you are prioritizing the neutral shape of your spine and not overextending. With a one-arm overhead press, you will press a dumbbell or kettlebell overhead in one hand while the other hand is unloaded. The unloaded hand can go on your side or out for balance. You can also use two different loads, with a lighter load on the weaker side at first. Eventually, the weaker side will catch up. The body has the ability to adapt using a phenomenon called cross-education. By training the right side, the left side gains strength, as well. This allows you to use a heavier load on the stronger side and still get the benefits for both sides.

2. **Single-Arm Chest Press:** Like the overhead press, you can use a lighter load on the weaker side. If you are on a bench or a stability ball while doing your chest press, you will need more core control because the load of the dumbbell can pull you to one side. Be mindful about being engaged and active in your core, which you can do by pressing your lower back down onto the bench. You should notice your core turn on. If you are on a stability ball, you'll want to bring your feet wider than shoulder width and squeeze your glutes to help control your pelvis, which will help with core activation.

3. **Renegade Row:** The chest press and overhead press are both pushing activities, but the renegade row is a pulling activity—one of my favorites. For those who sit hunched over a computer all day, you are typically weaker in the back and tighter in the front—weak back muscles and tight chest muscles. This is what gives you the hunched look. Strengthening your back muscles can help with posture. Doing single-sided renegade rows can help with shoulder and back imbalances from side to side. Grab a single dumbbell. Get into a high plank position. With the dumbbell in one hand and the other hand on the floor supporting you, row the dumbbell from the floor up to the side of your ribcage. Be mindful not to let your hips swivel, which would indicate a lack of core control. Squeeze your glutes and create as much stiffness as you can in your body to help support your spine.

Additional Assessments and Fixes

Squat Assessment and Fixes

As discussed in Chapter 3, the squat can be a great way to identify imbalances in the body. I explained how to assess a slow and controlled squat. You can also assess the squat using speed. By speeding up the movement, you can begin to see additional patterns of instability and imbalance.

First, do 10 squats slowly, making sure your toes are pointed forward, your heels stay on the ground, your back stays flat, the arch of your foot stays open, and your knees don't collapse inward. In a slow squat, you have the time to really connect to the movement, talking yourself through each aspect of stability as you go.

Now, let's add speed. You might try squatting as fast as possible—up down, up down, up down, like in the Swiss 1-Minute Sit-to-Stand Test from the fitness check-up. Or you might try doing a squat jump: you squat, jump, and land right back into your next squat jump, one right after the other. These fast squats are more difficult to connect to, and thus, allow a better way to see imbalances. Set up your phone to record again and try the speed squat 10 times fast or the squat jump 10 times fast. When you watch the video, you may notice imbalances you didn't see when you were doing slow, connected squats.

Things to look for:

Toes Turn Out in Squat

Squatting is a multi-joint movement, so there is a lot going on. Look first at your feet. Are your toes pointing forward? Or is one foot forward and one foot pointing out to the side while squatting? When the toes are pointed out in a duck-footed manner, it can mean several things, but most often it means you are missing internal range of motion in flexion at the hip. This creates pressure on the ACL and MCL in the knee, which is not sustainable and will lead to injury. The following two stretches can help mobilize the hips and improve hip range of motion:

Wall Internal Rotation Stretch

1. Lie down on your back with your feet flat against a wall so your hips and knees are at 90 degrees. Your hips will be on the floor.
2. Take your left foot and cross it over your right knee and use it to gently push your right knee in toward the midline of your body. Make sure your hips stay on the ground. Hold for up to two minutes and then switch sides.
3. If you feel pinching in your hip as you do this, use your hands to press down on the knee on that same side (as if you are pressing

it into the hip socket). The pinching in the hip is usually due to lack of range of motion in that joint. This stretch will help.

Shin-to-Wall Stretch

Ideally in a squat, if you were to draw a line from the angle of your torso and another line from the angle of your shin, those lines should never intersect. If they do, this means you likely have tight hip flexors that are pulling your torso forward, which can put quite a bit of stress on your lower back. Most of us are tight in the front of the hip, the hip flexors, from sitting too much. The shin-to-wall stretch, developed by physical therapist Dr. Kelly Starret, is great in helping to mobilize the hip.

1. Place your left knee on the floor against the wall, where the floor meets the wall. Your left shin will be against the wall.

2. Place your right foot flat on the floor in front of you, as if you are in a low lunge.

3. If you feel a deep stretch in the front of your left hip, hold there with two hands on the floor inside your right foot.

4. If you want to take it up a level, take your hands off the floor and raise your torso so it is parallel to the wall behind you. Actively squeeze your glute of the left leg and hold for up to two minutes, then switch sides. (At first you might not be able to do this, so take it slow.)

Just like foam rolling, for a stretch to be effective and change tissue, there may be some discomfort. You don't want it to be painful, but discomfort is okay. You may get some relief if you are tight by doing some of these mobilizations, but to see a long-term change, you must continue to work on these daily.

Arch of Foot Collapses in the Squat

Watch your squat video and look at the arches of your feet as you squat. Are they collapsed inward? If your arch collapses, your feet will turn out and your knees will collapse inward as described above. It's important to have an open arch, even for those who are more flat-footed. The arch helps our joints absorb the shock of landing in a walk or run. If the arch is not open, that can lead to shin splints, knee pain, and hip issues because you are missing that first level of force absorption in your foot and all the force of landing on a walking or running step goes into the shin, knee, and hip. The arch was designed to handle that load and make it easier on our other joints. As described in Chapter 3, you can actively create arches in your foot. Take your big toe and heel and push them down on the floor. Keeping your knees locked out, tear the ground apart with your feet. Imagine standing on a piece of paper and trying to rip it down the middle using your feet. Your knees will rotate out slightly, your femur will rotate out, and your arches will open up. You should feel torque under your feet.

Notice that you must use your glutes to do this. When your glutes are activated, you're creating stability around your hips. This stability will allow you to be strong as you squat. For some of you who are hypermobile or have a lot of flexibility, it can be hard to create stability like this. See below for more information about hypermobility.

Heels Lift up in a Squat

If you look at the profile view of your squat, watch to ensure that your heels don't come off the floor. If they do, the ankle isn't allowing the shin to go forward, so the only way you can squat is to pick the heel up. Or you might turn your toes out to work your way around the missing range of motion at your ankles. Either way, this creates a shear force on the knee, which isn't good. A shear force is when unaligned forces act on a joint. The shearing on a joint can wear away at the tissue designed to keep the joint healthy and mobile. One of the ways to increase the range of motion at your ankle is to do this simple **ankle mobility exercise**:

1. Drop down into a lunge position with your left knee on the floor under your hips and your right foot flat on the floor in front of you.
2. You will anchor your heel to the ground with your right hand by pushing from your achilles into your heel so you make sure the heel stays on the floor.
3. Then lean forward, place your left hand on your knee, and push your knee forward as far over your toes as possible. Hold for up to two minutes and then switch sides.
4. The key is to make sure that the ankle stays right in the middle of the foot and doesn't wobble side to side. You'll notice when the ankle collapses in, so does the arch of the foot and so does the knee. It's important to keep the arch of the foot open. If you want to ramp this up, you can set a kettlebell or dumbbell on your knee and use that as an additional load to move your knee forward.

Overhead Press Fixes—Upper Back and Shoulder Mobilization

When you have upper back stiffness, your lower back or shoulders will compensate. If you were missing range of motion in your overhead assessment and couldn't get your arms overhead, you probably noticed that if you let your rib cage open and arch the lower back, you could get your thumbs to touch the ground overhead with your elbows locked out. That is not safe. Imagine standing up in that same position, holding a dumbbell over your head, with your rib cage open and your lower back arched. All those vertebrae in your lower back are compressed and at high risk of injury.

One of the things I like to do when thinking of restoring range of motion to a position is to find ways to express that same position under restriction. In other words, your upper back and shoulders are stiff, and you must arch your lower back to get your arms overhead. Can we find a way to get you in the overhead position without arching your lower back but working on undoing the stiffness in your shoulders and upper back? Yes, and you'll need a foam roller and a kettlebell or something to use as an anchor.

1. Lie on the ground on your back. Take a foam roller under your upper back at a 90-degree angle so it intersects your upper back. Start with it between your shoulder blades.

2. Make sure the kettlebell, or whatever you're using as an anchor, is above your head on the floor.

3. Keeping your feet flat on the ground with your knees bent, press your hips up.

4. Grab the kettlebell that is overhead with both hands while keeping the foam roller under your upper back. Make sure your arms are still and elbows locked out.

5. Very important now to be strong in your core and brace like you are taking a punch to the stomach. While doing this and keeping your elbows locked out, slowly lower your hips to the ground. Repeat raising and lowering your hips for up to two minutes. Then find another spot on your upper back to try and loosen using the same technique.

Hanging from a bar and breathing also helps build some space between vertebrae and can help unglue the shoulders and upper back. You don't have to hang with your full body weight if that's too much; you could put a foot up on a box or bench and hang with a little body weight, but the loaded hanging will help open up some of the tissue that might be tight, and the breathing will help you expand the ribcage and give you more mobility in your upper back.

APPENDIX C

Hypermobility, Isometric Exercises, Eccentric Training, and Instability

As mentioned in Chapter 3, hypermobility is when you have beyond normal range of motion around joints. In other words, you can move some or all of your joints past what most people can. Simply said, you may be very flexible. Sometimes with hypermobility comes looseness or slack in the joints. Looseness in muscles and tendons usually means long and weak, while tight means strong and overactive. Both are associated with an increased risk of injury. Hypermobility can create issues when it comes to strength training.

The hypermobile person is often unfamiliar with the feeling of creating stability and stiffness in the system and around joints. Look back to the squat and remember how you create stability by using your feet. This concept of stability, of grinding through a range of motion like a squat or a push-up, is a challenging concept to understand and feel when you are loose and hypermobile. I like to use isometric exercises and eccentric negatives to teach someone who is hypermobile how to create stability. Learning to be stable in different positions allows you to own a position and be strong in that position, as opposed to just hanging out in that position.

Isometric Activities

Isometric is a way to train that doesn't allow you to move; you just hold a position. I like these for the hypermobile person because you don't have to worry about staying connected to a position as you move through it; you can just hold it and focus on that one position.

High planks are a great isometric exercise. The high plank, which is the top of your push-up, gives you the skill of using your hands, just like you use your feet in the squat, to create stability—tearing at the floor with your hands to create torque under your hands so the eye of your elbow is facing forward and your hands are actively gripping at the floor. This creates stability at the shoulder. Using glutes to stabilize your pelvis and organize your spine by engaging your core and bracing will create intentional stability, as well. You can scale this up by also holding in the bottom of the push-up with the chest just a few inches off the ground.

The same works for a **squat**. Hold the bottom position of a squat and go over your checklist: toes forward, big toe and heel down, arch of foot open, knees driving out laterally, back flat. You can try holding at different depths. How long? Until it burns and then a few more seconds. Again, the key is to own the shape, not just hang out. Be stiff, feel tension under your feet or your hands, and organize your spine.

You can also do this with a **lunge** by holding with the back knee just right off the floor. You can do isometrics with barbells and dumbbells. Try holding a barbell overhead using the cues in the overhead assessment. Go until you start to shake, then just hold on a bit more and then rest.

Eccentric Training

Eccentric movement refers to the part of any movement in which the muscle fibers are pulling apart or lengthening. It's sometimes known as the negative part of movement. In a push-up, the eccentric is on the way down. The opposite is the concentric, which is on the way up. For the squat, eccentric is on the way down, concentric is on the way up. We are always stronger when we move eccentrically. You could put a heavy barbell on your back and squat down, but getting up would be much harder. The way down on a push-up is much easier than the way up.

The way eccentrics work is to slow down the tempo of your movement on the eccentric part of an exercise. Since you are stronger during this part of the movement, you can slow it down more easily and use the cues you know to create stability to connect to the movement. Try doing push-ups with a three count on the way down while using your hands to create stability at the shoulder, as described in the previous section. Lower your body, keeping your hip and shoulder connected and moving simultaneously through a stiff spine. Once you get to the bottom, see if you can push your way back up, but with no restriction on the tempo. If you must put your knees on the ground to get back up, that's okay. It's a great place to start...lowering down slowly on your feet in a high plank and then setting your knees down to press back up. How many? Until you are shaking, then do one more. You can do the same with the squat. Think of the stability cues for the squat and lower down slowly while you focus and grind, then return to the top. If you want to be further challenged, you can do a 1¼ rep. Go slow in the squat or push-up on the way down. Once you hit the bottom, come up only a quarter of the way, lower back down slowly, and then come up. I like this because it provides more time under tension, which forces you to own the position at each change and all along the way.

Instability

I also like to use instability to help force stability, to put someone in an unstable environment to help them understand how to create stability. I use wobble boards, BOSU balls, stability balls, and foam pads to create instability. For most hypermobile people or those who don't have a good concept of stability, just having them stand on a foam pad or a BOSU ball can be challenging because they almost shake right off the BOSU ball or wobble board. With the right cues of stability, toes forward, knees out, or hands gripping, back flat, you can start to take back some control of the shaky, unstable feeling you get when in an unstable situation.

To try this, first squat on a BOSU or wobble board, then squat on the floor using the same stability cues. You'll notice how the skill of stability transfers from unstable to stable. If you don't have a BOSU or wobble board, you can close your eyes and squat or try to balance on one foot with your eyes closed. You use your vision to help create stability through proprioception. Taking your vision away will challenge you to rely more on your ability to find stability using cues like the ones we have gone over above.

Here is a list of activities to get you thinking about how to use unstable environments to help create stability:

1. Push-ups with shoulder taps: Do a push-up, and then at the top, balance on one hand as you tap the opposite shoulder. Then switch hands. Don't just do it; think about how you must use your supporting hand to grip the floor and create stability. Be sure to tighten around the spine and pelvis to prevent the hips from shifting side to side.

2. Front-loaded squats on BOSU: Hold dumbbells or a kettle-bell in front of you close to your body, and use the squatting technique while you perform squats on a BOSU ball. It will force you to slow down and think about how to stay connected and create stability.

3. Plank on a stability ball: Try holding a plank with hands on the stability ball and feet on the ground, using the cues to create stability at the shoulder, pelvis, and spine. If you want to make this even more challenging, try to do a push-up, with hands on the stability ball and feet on the ground. Ensure you grip the ball on the sides with your fingertips pointing down.

APPENDIX D
Mobility for Sitting Too Much

As discussed in Chapter 8, sitting too long can increase your risk of soft tissue injuries and cause imbalances in your body. The most common imbalances are being short and tight in the front of the hip and shoulders and weak in the back of the legs and back. In general, to help begin to reverse the effects of sitting, you want to find ways to stretch the front and strengthen the back of your body. Here are some activities that might help with balancing your body:

1. Shin-to-wall stretch (directions on pg. 199)
2. Glute activation: A simple way to activate the glutes is by doing side-lying leg lifts. Lying on your side, with a stiff leg and locked knee, bring your top leg away from the midline of your body and then slightly behind you. Start by holding it here for 5 to 10 seconds and seeing if you can feel your glute working. Make sure you're keeping your core engaged and not collapsing into the ribs that are on the floor.

3. Chest stretch and upper back activation: For the chest stretch, lie down on a foam roller so the roller is parallel to your spine. Make sure your head and shoulders are supported on the foam roller. Place your fingertips behind your ears and actively drive your elbows toward the ground as you stretch your chest.

4. Upper back strengthening with a band pull-apart: I like to use a resistance band while standing against the wall with the hips, shoulders, and back of the head on the wall. With one end of the band in each hand, pull the band as far apart as you can. Make sure to keep the head, shoulders, and hips in contact with the wall the entire time.

If you don't have the option of standing more and sitting less, you can try the following to mitigate the risk of soft tissue injury and imbalances that come with sitting for more than six hours a day:

1. Before you sit for a longer period, do the shin-to-wall stretch for a couple of minutes on each side. This will stretch the front of your legs, which get chronically short with too much sitting.

2. Foam roll on your I.T. bands, which are on the outside of your legs from hip to knee. Also, roll on your quads, the front of your legs from hip to knee. This tissue can also get short and tight with too much sitting.

3. Do the best you can to get up and move around, even if just for a couple of minutes each hour.

4. Make sure that when you are sitting, you are sitting with good posture.

APPENDIX E

Carb Cycling and Nutrition Resources

Carb cycling is the term used for cycling through lower and higher carbohydrate days to support health, weight loss, energy, and lifestyle. I find this to be a sustainable alternative to extreme carb restriction, and it yields the same healthy benefits but in a way that supports most lifestyles.

We need carbohydrates as fuel to perform. More nutrient-dense carbohydrates like vegetables and fruits give us more sustainable energy for longer periods of time. When eating carbs, focus on whole foods like fruits, vegetables, and whole grains. Highly processed carbohydrates like crackers, cookies, and highly processed breads give us a higher spike in blood sugar and energy and then get stored as fat.

Low-carb dieting has been around since the 1970s, but was made popular in the 1990s by Dr. Atkins in his *New Diet Revolution*. Low-carb dieting works to lose weight, but it's generally not sustainable, and the older we get and the more active we become, the more we need healthy carbs to balance our nutrition with the energy required to train. Carb cycling is a way to try and get that balance by cycling high-carb days with high-intensity training days and lower-carb days with lower-intensity training days. Carbs become the fuel we need to train hard, as in short, aggressive cardio intervals and high-intensity training. The rub is that if we eat carbs and don't follow it with hard training, that energy converts to fat.

You don't have to be strict about this. Maybe you went out to dinner or had more carbohydrates than you typically do. The next day, you can simply restrict carbohydrates a little. It can be that simple, and is an option for those who want weight loss to be part of your practice.

Limiting carbs can be a tool for weight loss because carbs that aren't converted to sugar in the blood are stored as fat in the body. The only way to ensure that we use the carbs converted to sugar is to move. If we eat too many carbs or don't move enough, those carbs go from sugar in the blood to fat in the body. Highly processed carbs get stored as fat much more quickly because they spike glucose fast and only give you a small window to use them as energy. Limiting carbs to the point of starvation or even excess hunger will force the body to hold on to fat.

In general, for any training over 80 percent intensity, you can consume about twice the amount of carbs compared to your lower carb days. For this to work, you have to go back to the adaptation cycle and make sure the stimulus is strong enough to cause fatigue. You will burn more carbs on high-intensity anaerobic training days. In order to be able to push yourself hard enough you **need** to have those carbs available on those days. This cycling system of lower carbs on less-demanding training days and higher carbs on more intense days will give you the energy to train harder when you want to and also have the benefits of some weight loss when you are not training as hard. Remember, this isn't all about weight loss. High-intensity training is also about antiaging and hormone production, so those challenging training days have to be fueled properly.

Constantly adjust and experiment with what works for you. On certain training days, for example, if it's a longer, harder interval running day, you may need more carbs to feel better and perform better. On easier days, such as a recovery hike or walk, you can experiment with lower carbs.

Once you have done the initial work to determine the number of carbs in most foods you eat, you will no longer have to track everything and add up your carbs. However, I recommend doing this for the first week until you get the idea. (~25 grams of carbs in 1 apple, ~50 grams of carbs in a bagel, ~ 2 grams of carbs in coffee creamer, etc.)

When talking about carbs, I'm talking about total carbs, not net carbs. Net carbs are calculated by subtracting fiber or sugar alcohol from the label. Technically, net carbs are the carbs the body can absorb because the fiber and sugar alcohols aren't absorbed and turned into glucose or energy. The net and total carbs don't matter, especially if you eat mostly whole foods.

How to get started

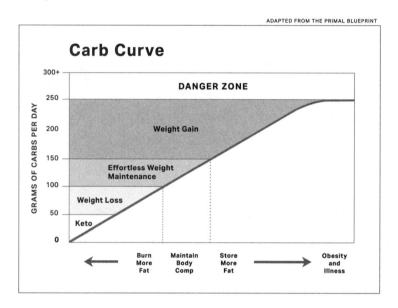

As you look at the carb graph you can see where weight loss starts to occur in most people. Again, we are all different, so we will all respond differently to different levels of high and low carb intake. A good place to start is to take a look at your food journal that I was talking about before. Calculate on average how many carbs you have in a day. Maybe start 50–100 grams lower than what you normally do for a low carb day. Don't rush from 200 grams to 50 grams. The key is finding a sweet spot that is sustainable. I recommend being patient to see how you feel and if you are getting the results you want. This may take a week or two.

Try each one for at least a week. Track weight, energy levels, and how well you felt like you performed in workouts. It's important to feel good and have energy on high-intensity training days. Decide what works for you and cycle through the days of restricting carbs with easier workouts and then allowing more carbs on hard training days. It's different for everyone, but depending on how hard you are training, you may end up doubling your carbs from your low days to your high days. This is if you are really low on low days, 50–100 grams or less, and training really hard on high days.

Some people live in this cycling state, and it works. Not everyone is exact, and as a matter of fact, most people, once they figure it out, just kind of ebb and flow because they know what works for them. They don't go around all day counting every carb. That's not sustainable.

The actual timing of when to consume your carbs on higher-intensity training days will depend on when you are training. Ideally, you would have more carbs before you train. If you train early, this might mean having something you can tolerate before training. Typically something lower in fiber and fat because fiber and fat are harder to digest and can cause abdominal cramping if consumed too close to training. It could be a smoothie with berries, a banana, and a milk alternative. It could also be adding some electrolytes and carbs to your water bottle. But note that many sports drinks can cause gastrointestinal issues because of the different types of sugars in them that are not easily digested. Watch out for sucrose, maltodextrin, and high fructose corn syrup.

The National Council on Sports Medicine recommends about 1 gram of carbs per kilogram of body weight about 1 hour before your workout for longer, harder training sessions. To have the carbohydrates available for performance, you want to consume them early enough. It's also okay to have your additional carbs the night before your high-intensity training session. I like to do that and then have additional carbs after the workout to support recovery. You'll learn what feels best for you and know that carb cycling isn't for everyone. If it's not for you, don't do it.

Resources for Nutrition

Paleo Running Mama

https://www.paleorunningmomma.com/

Half Baked Harvest

https://www.halfbakedharvest.com/recipes/

Blue Zones

https://www.bluezones.com/recipes/

Well Plated

https://www.wellplated.com/

Cookie and Kate

https://cookieandkate.com/

Higher-Level Fitness Tests

After being around fitness for so many years, I have found a few simple measurables that can provide instant feedback for the average fitness enthusiast. The following aren't the well-researched fitness standards I use for the fitness check-up, but they are good measures of fitness for the average gym enthusiast. If squats, push-ups, burpees, and simple kettlebell bell movements are in your repertoire, I recommend trying these three fitness levels to see if you can pass each. In our studio, we offer this test a few times a year, and our pass rate for all three levels is close to 90 percent for clients who have been with us for three months or more.

These three short workouts use higher intensity training using shorter interval-style efforts. Most people are much more accustomed to longer efforts of cardio or exercise, but when asked to increase intensity to something higher and not as sustainable, they run into serious deficiencies. Ready to try these?

Test 1

Can you complete two rounds of the following work in 4 minutes?

- 10 push-ups (release your hands from the floor in the bottom position of the push-up, just like the hand-release push-up test in the fitness check-up)
- 15 air squats (touch your butt to a chair or target at about knee height, just like in the sit-to-stand test)
- 5 burpees (however you want to get down to the floor and then push your body weight off the floor and stand back up)

If you can do this, try the next one. If you ran into problems on the first test, it might be a sign that you are deconditioned, or if you were limited by pain or discomfort, it also might be a sign that you need some help with movement. A good place to start would be going back to the fitness check-up and seeing what your lowest score was, and trying to work on those weaknesses.

Test 2

Can you complete two rounds of the following work in 6 minutes?

- .25 mile (400 meters) run, walk, jog, or on a rowing machine
- 20 total step-ups to a bench or chair at about knee height (do 10 in a row on each side)

If this one went well for you, move on to the next test. If not, I would assess what your limitations were on this. Was it the amount of work? Was the cardiovascular part too much or was it the strength work? Or maybe a combination of both? Again, if your limiting factor was pain or discomfort in joints or muscles, remember that you need to bring some awareness into how you are moving and what might be missing so you can try on your own to solve problems like a tight hamstring or a weak lower back.

Test 3

* For this test, you will need a kettlebell that would be challenging to swing overhead 40–50 times in a row. If you have made it this far, you should own or have access to a kettlebell. If not, consider purchasing one. You can do a lot with just a single kettlebell at home.

Can you complete the following work in 20 minutes?

- 800 meters or .50 mile
- 30 kettlebell swings overhead: Swing the kettlebell from between the knees to overhead.
- 30 front squats holding the same load kettlebell: Hold the kettlebell under the chin as you squat.
- 30 kettlebell swings overhead
- 30 total lunge steps holding the same load kettlebell: Again, hold the kettlebell under the chin as you lunge, alternating either forward or backward for each lunge step.
- 800 meters
- 20 kettlebell high pull: Start with the kettlebell on the floor. Squat down to pick up the kettlebell with both hands and then as you stand pull the kettlebell under the chin as you drive your elbows high to the ceiling.

- 20 sprawl: Do a burpee but with no push-up.
- 20 kettlebell high pull
- 20 burpees: This burpee will need a push-up where your chest touches the floor each time.
- 800 meters or .50 mile

If you passed this last test in time, congratulations! If not, don't worry; it's just information for you, and these aren't the only ways to test fitness. These are three simple tests that work inside my world of fitness that I thought I would share with you.

APPENDIX G
Specific Exercises to Improve Your Fit Score

How to Improve Sit-to-Rise Score

Mobility:

- Pigeon pose
- Seated windshield wiper pose
- Develop a good yoga practice

Strength:

Narrow squat from the floor. To do this, start seated on the floor with your feet in front of you and knees bent. If you can't stand up without using your hands, then have something to hold onto that is in front of you, such as an exercise band around something like a heavy table leg. Then, use the band to help support you in getting up. If you don't have a band, you can just use something stationary anchored to the floor and close to your body.

- Single leg squats to as deep a target as you can control the squat. Keep lowering your target as you get stronger.

How to Improve Dead Hang Score

Strength:

- Heavy farmer's carry: Hold a kettlebell or dumbbell in each hand. Make it as heavy as you can. Walk as far as you can, holding the dumbbells. Go until your grip fails, then set the dumbbells down and rest. Repeat 5–10 more sets.
- TRX pull-ups (Any suspended training system will work for this. The TRX are straps that hang from the ceiling, a door, or any anchor above your head. Most suspended trainers come with two handles to hold onto as you pull your body up.)
- Kettlebell swings
- Dead hang from a bar

How to Improve 1-minute Sit-to-Stand Score

Basic-Level Squat Workout:

Complete as many rounds of the following until you fatigue. Stop before your movement mechanics fail due to fatigue.

- Ten squats to an 18-inch surface
- Ten static lunge steps per side (just going up and down, your feet don't leave the ground)
- 30 seconds of high plank

Moderate-Level Squat Workout:

Complete at least three rounds of the following work. This should be challenging and feel like work. Once you fatigue, rest and do one more round.

- 10 squats to touch your butt to an 18-inch surface

- 10 light squat jumps to touch your butt to an 18-inch surface
- 10 static lunge steps per side
- 30 seconds of high to low plank (keeping hip stable transition back and forth from hands to forearms)

Advanced-Level Squat Workout:

Complete at least four rounds of the following work. This should be challenging and feel like work. Once you can no longer complete the required work in a minute, you are done.

You have 1 minute to complete the following work and then 1 minute to rest—and *yes*, you are doing all this work in 60 seconds:

- 10 squats to touch your butt to an 18-inch surface
- 10 light squat jumps to touch your butt to an 18-inch surface
- 10 lunge steps total, alternating sides
- 10 lunge jumps total (from the bottom of your lunge, jump and switch your feet in the air to land back in the lunge position)

If you want this to be very challenging, hold a 1-minute plank during your rest.

Higher Level Loaded Squat Activities:

- Back squats
- Front squats
- Deadlifts
- Loaded lunge steps

How to Improve Air Force 2-minute Hand-Release Push-up Test

Basic-Level Upper Body Workout:

Complete as many rounds of the following until you fatigue. Stop before your movement mechanics fail due to fatigue.

- 5–10 push-ups on an incline (hands on chair or bench, feet or knees on the ground)
- 5–10 TRX pull-ups (any suspended trainer will work)
- 30 seconds wall sit

Moderate-Level Upper Body Workout:

Complete at least three rounds of the following work. This should be challenging and feel like work. Once you fatigue, rest and do one more round.

- 3 narrow push-ups with hands inside shoulders. Knees or feet on the floor. Chest to the floor with each repetition.
- 4 wide push-ups with hands outside shoulders. Knees or feet on the floor. Chest to the floor with each repetition.
- 5 regular push-ups with the hands under the shoulders. Knees or feet on the floor. Chest to the floor with each repetition.
- 30 seconds of as many squats as you can do to an 18-inch surface.

*If you want to make this more challenging, try transitioning from one push-up type to the next without resting. On the other hand, if you can't do push-ups with feet on floor, you can switch to knees on floor.

Advanced-Level Upper Body Workout:
Complete at least four rounds of the following work. This should be challenging and feel like work. Once you can no longer complete the required work in a minute, you are done.

You have 1 minute to complete the work and then 1 minute to rest:

- 5 hand-release push-ups
- 4 burpees (complete a full hand-release push-up in the bottom of your burpee)
- 3 double push-up burpees (complete two full hand-release push-ups in the bottom of your burpee)

If you want to make this more challenging, hold a 1-minute wall sit during your rest. If you want this to be even more challenging, add one hand-release push-up at the top of each round. Example round 2: 6 hand-release push-ups, 4 burpees, 3 double push-up burpees.

Higher-Level Loaded Upper Body Activities
- Chest press
- Overhead press
- Pull-ups or TRX pull-ups
- Dumbbell or barbell bent rows

How to Improve 1-Mile Time

Basic Level 1 Cardio Workout:

Complete as many rounds of the following until you fatigue. A good goal to start is three efforts, building to five efforts. Take your 1-mile pace and go 30–60 seconds faster for this workout.

- 2 minutes at 30–60 seconds faster than 1-mile pace, 2 minutes active rest (this could be a light jog or walk)

Moderate-Level Cardio Workout:

Complete as many rounds of the following until you fatigue. A good goal to start is five efforts, building to 10 efforts. Take your 1-mile pace and go 45–75 seconds faster for this workout.

- 1 minute at 45–75 seconds faster than 1-mile pace, 2 minutes active rest (this could be a light jog or walk)

Advanced-Level Cardio Workout:

Complete as many rounds of the following until you fatigue. A good goal to start is 15 efforts, building to 30 efforts. Take your 1-mile pace and go 90–120 seconds faster for this workout

- 30 seconds at 90–120 seconds faster than 1-mile pace, 90 seconds active rest (this could be a light jog or walk)

If you want this to be even more challenging, add 2–5 burpees during each 90-second rest period.

Additional (Fun!) Challenges

Burpee Challenge

Start standing to full push-up, chest to floor, then back to full standing.

- Gold = 24+ burpees in 1 minute
- Silver = 18+ burpees in 1 minute
- Bronze = 15+ burpees in 1 minute

Mixed Element Challenge

Find a kettlebell that you can swing to shoulder level about 30 times but not 40 times.

Complete five rounds of the following in less than 15 minutes:

- 25 kettlebell swings to shoulder level (Russian style)
- 20 air squats
- 10 burpees (chest to floor each time)

If you want to make this more challenging, hold your kettlebell in front of your chest under your chin while you do the squats.

Broken Mile Challenge

Your goal is to run everything at or faster than your fitness check-up 1-mile time. You are allowed to rest for the same amount of time you worked after each effort and between the .25 mile and .50 mile efforts.

- 4 x .25 mile (Rest after each effort for the same amount of time that you worked.)
- 2 x .50 mile (Rest after each effort for the same amount of time that you worked.)
- 1 x 1 mile

This work can be done on a treadmill, track, or a rowing machine.

Citations

1. Ages of 40–59 you will gain more weight than any other point in your life. https://www.cdc.gov/obesity/data/adult.html

2. When we reach 40 years old, the production of sex hormones begins to decrease by up to 3% per year. https://www.ncbi.nlm.nih.gov/pmc/articles/PMC3636678/

3. Needle procedures related fear may result in increased avoidance behavior and attempt to eliminate any exposure to needles. https://www.ncbi.nlm.nih.gov/pmc/articles/PMC7774419/

4. Moving puts you in the top 17% of the U.S. population for your age. https://www.medicalnewstoday.com/articles/fitness-routines-after-40#:~:text=That%20number%20increased%20to%2017.2,both%20physical%20and%20cognitive%20decline.

5. Male testosterone drops on average 3% per year after the age of 40. https://clevelandurology.net/posts/mens-health/when-do-men-need-low-testosterone-treatment/#:~:text=A%20man's%20ability%20to%20produce,men%20are%20candidates%20for%20therapy.

6. Estrogen peaks in late 20s and drops 50% by the age of 50. https://www.verywellhealth.com/low-estrogen-levels-4588661#:~:text=A%20woman's%20estrogen%20levels%20peak,consecutive%20months%20without%20a%20period.

7. Women as early as 30 will see a 3–5% lean muscle loss per year. https://www.henryford.com/blog/2023/01/how-to-maintain-muscle-mass-as-you-age#:~:text=As%20we%20age%20it's%20 normal,rebuild%20muscle%20at%20any%20age.

8. York University treadmill study on intensity. https://www.ncbi.nlm. nih.gov/pmc/articles/PMC4024007/

9. 78% of people who train for a marathon don't lose or gain weight. https://www.thecut.com/2015/10/on-the-mysteries-of-marathon-weight-gain.html

10. You need a minimum of 8 hours of sleep in order to get 25% in deep sleep. https://www.healthline.com/health/how-much-deep-sleep-do-you-need#:~:text=Deep%20sleep%20is%20essential%20for,this%20 should%20be%20deep%20sleep.

11. Collagen decreases joint pain and increases recovery time with 10 gram dose daily. https://www.ncbi.nlm.nih.gov/pmc/articles/ PMC10058045/#:~:text=Using%20another%20hydrolyzed%20 collagen%2C%20Benito,high%20variability%20in%20 administration%20time.

12. 10% imbalance in muscle strength can lead to increased risk of injury. https://www.mendcolorado.com/physical-therapy-blog/2019/12/7/ impact-of-lower-body-muscle-imbalances-on-performance-and-injury-risk/#:~:text=Previous%20authors%20have%20found%20 a,the%20validity%20of%20this%20number.

13. Studies show us that sitting is closely related to nerve desensitization. https://lluh.org/services/neuropathic-therapy-center/blog/5-ways-sitting-killing-your-nerves#:~:text=The%20longer%20one%20 sits%2C%20the,tingling%2C%20burning%20or%20stabbing%20pain.

14. According to Healthline, sitting on the floor leads to "natural stability." https://www.healthline.com/health/sitting-on-the-floor#:~:text=The%20practice%20is%20said%20to,if%20already%20 have%20joint%20issues.

15. At the age of 50 we start losing more bone density than we can produce. Some women can lose up to 20% within 5–7 years following menopause. https://www.bonehealthandosteoporosis. org/preventing-fractures/general-facts/what-women-need-to-know/#:~:text=How%20fast%20you%20lose%20bone,greater%20 chance%20of%20developing%20osteoporosis.

16. 73% of people who start a fitness program quit because the program is too challenging, boring, or ineffective. https:// www.businesswire.com/news/home/20121226005078/en/ New-Study-Finds-73-Percent-of-People-Who-Set-Fitness-Goals-as-New-Year%E2%80%99s-Resolutions-Give-Them-Up

17. Sit-to-Rise Study. https://pubmed.ncbi.nlm.nih.gov/23242910/

18. Grip strength and DNA age acceleration study. https://pubmed.ncbi. nlm.nih.gov/36353822/

19 Study on grip strength 50–65 years old from Tobago. https://www. ncbi.nlm.nih.gov/pmc/articles/PMC3335373/

20. Study published in the NLM in 2022, men averaged a grip force of 48 KG while women averaged 33 KG. https://www.ncbi.nlm. nih.gov/pmc/articles/PMC8995759/#:~:text=The%20maximal%20 handgrip%20strength%20was,67.7%25%20of%20that%20of%20males

21. Switzerland one of the top four countries in life expectancy. https:// www.worldometers.info/demographics/life-expectancy/

22. Swiss Sit to Stand Study. https://igptr.ch/wp-content/ uploads/2023/04/2013_Strassmann-A_Population-based-reference-values-for-the-1-min-sit-to-stand-test.pdf

23. Meta-analysis related to lower body strength endurance showed that those with above-average lower body strength endurance had a 14% lower risk of death. https://pubmed.ncbi.nlm.nih.gov/29425700/

24. In a 44-year study on 2,000 people published in the NLM, those with better upper body strength live longer and have a later onset of disease. https://www.ncbi.nlm.nih.gov/pmc/articles/PMC3337929/

25. In January 2022, the U.S. Air Force released its new push-up test. https://www.airandspaceforces.com/article/ here-are-the-scoring-charts-for-the-air-forces-new-pt-test-exercises- minus-the-walk/#:~:text=Hand%2Drelease%20pushups%20are%20 scored,30%20to%2040%20or%20more.

26. General CQ Brown Jr. said, "We are moving away from a one-size-fits-all model." https://barbell-logic.com/military- physical-readiness/#:~:text=General%20Charles%20 Q.,Airmen%E2%80%94where%20it%20belongs.%E2%80%9D

27. The Rand Corporation found that less than 1% of U.S. airmen and airwomen are at risk of adverse health conditions. https://www.rand. org/pubs/research_reports/RRA552-1.html

28. 20% of Air Force is made up of women pilots and officers. https:// www.zippia.com/air-force-pilot-jobs/demographics/

29. A 55-year-old man who can cover a mile in 15 minutes has a 30% chance of developing heart disease. https://www.sciencedaily. com/releases/2011/05/110518121229.htm#:~:text=For%20 example%2C%20a%2055%2Dyear,of%20less%20than%2010%20 percent

30. Running Level 1 mile run times. https://runninglevel.com/ running-times/1-mile-times

31. Wall Sit Norms. https://foundationchiropractic.ca/ at-home-fitness-testing/

32. Plank Hold Norms. https://www.topendsports.com/testing/tests/ plank.htm

33. 2 KM Rowing Norms. https://rowinglevel.com/ rowing-times/2000m-times

34. Dan Buettner "high quality of life in their old age." https:// itsthyme2cook.com/traditional-minestrone-with-a- twist/#:~:text=The%20term%20%E2%80%9CBlue%20 Zone%E2%80%9D%20was,is%20one%20of%20those%20regions.

35. "Centenarians in all 5 blue zone areas enjoy much lower rates of chronic disease...." https://www.bluezones.com/meal-planner/#section-2

36. "Live in environments that constantly nudge them..." https://www.bchd.org/power-9-principles#:~:text=MOVE%20NATURALLY,house%20or%20places%20of%20worship.

37. Calories burned 13% in hard workout. https://www.health.harvard.edu/diet-and-weight-loss/calories-burned-in-30-minutes-for-people-of-three-different-weights

38. Calories burned by N.E.A.T. https://www.foodspring.co.uk/magazine/how-to-increase-neat#:~:text=Moving%20more%20throughout%20your%20daily,higher%20your%20total%20calorie%20needs.

39. A study published in the JLM found that for each daily 2-hour increment of sitting the risk of diabetes and obesity went up 5% and 7%, respectively. https://www.ncbi.nlm.nih.gov/pmc/articles/PMC5618737/

40. 2013 WHO estimated that 3.2 million people died prematurely from a sedentary lifestyle. https://www.who.int/data/gho/indicator-metadata-registry/imr-details/3416#:~:text=People%20who%20are%20insufficiently%20physically,of%20the%20week%20(10)

41. You are low-risk if you sit for less than 4 hours daily. https://www.juststand.org/the-tools/sitting-time-calculator/

42. Sitting for more than 8 hours is sedentary. https://www.mayoclinic.org/healthy-lifestyle/adult-health/expert-answers/sitting/faq-20058005#:~:text=Researchers%20analyzed%2013%20studies%20of,posed%20by%20obesity%20and%20smoking

43. 60% of U.S. adults are sedentary. https://www.cdc.gov/nccdphp/sgr/adults.htm#:~:text=Top%20of%20Page-,Facts,are%20not%20active%20at%20all.

44. Sedentary people have a 20-30% higher risk of all-cause mortality. https://www.who.int/data/gho/indicator-metadata-registry/imr-details/3416#:~:text=People%20who%20are%20insufficiently%20physically,of%20the%20week%20(10).

45. Cleveland Clinic recommendations for melatonin dosage. https://health.clevelandclinic.org/melatonin-how-much-should-i-take-for-a-good-nights-rest/

46. BMJ correlation between processed food intake and coronary heart disease. https://www.bmj.com/content/365/bmj.l1451

47. EWG processed food and depression. https://www.ewg.org/news-insights/news/2023/09/new-study-finds-possible-link-between-ultra-processed-foods-and

48. Sugar Intake. https://www.ars.usda.gov/plains-area/gfnd/gfhnrc/docs/news-articles/2012/the-question-of-sugar/#:~:text=The%20average%20American%20eats%20(or,sugars%20per%20person%20each%20year.

49. CDC sugar recommendations. https://www.cdc.gov/nutrition/data-statistics/added-sugars.html#:~:text=Americans%202%20years%20and%20older,sugars%20(about%2012%20teaspoons)

50. Sardinian's sugar intake 50 grams. https://www.monaottum.com/2017/01/10/sardinia-italy-home-of-the-healthiest-and-longest-living-men/#:~:text=7%20to%2010%20%E2%80%93%203%20ounce,olive%20oil%20but%20also%20lard

51. Obesity rate in Sardinia. https://pubmed.ncbi.nlm.nih.gov/17615488/#:~:text=Main%20findings%3A%20The%20overall%20prevalence,a%20significant%20protection%20against%20obesity.

52. Obesity rate in the United States. https://frac.org/obesity-health/obesity-u-s-2#:~:text=The%20latest%20data%20indicate%20that,tend%20to%20increase%20with%20age

53. Study showing alcohol and effects on REM sleep. https://www.ncbi. nlm.nih.gov/pmc/articles/PMC5821259/

54. CDC recommends 2 drinks for men and 1 for women daily. https://www.cdc.gov/alcohol/fact-sheets/moderate-drinking. htm#:~:text=To%20reduce%20the%20risk%20of,days%20when%20 alcohol%20is%20consumed

55. U.S. unhealthiest country in the world. https:// worldpopulationreview.com/country-rankings/ unhealthiest-country-in-the-world

56. WHO "no level of alcohol consumption is safe for our health." https://www.who.int/europe/news/item/04-01-2023-no-level-of-alcohol-consumption-is-safe-for-our-health#:~:text=The%20 World%20Health%20Organization%20has,that%20does%20not%20 affect%20health

57. Ketones' anti-seizure effect on the brain. https://www.ncbi.nlm.nih. gov/pmc/articles/PMC5771386/#:~:text=Ketone%20metabolism%20 gradually%20reduces%20neuronal,antiepileptic%20effects%20of%20 the%20KD

58. 800-gram challenge. https://optimizemenutrition.com/800g-challenge/#:~:text=I'm%20EC%20Synkowski%2C%20 creator,eliminating%20the%20foods%20you%20love!

59. Ideal body fat % for women 40–59 is 23–33% and for men 11–22%. https://www.webmd.com/fitness-exercise/what-is-body-composition

60. Study showing link between lean muscle and longevity. https://www. ncbi.nlm.nih.gov/pmc/articles/PMC4035379/

61. Intermittent fasting and longevity study. https:// zerolongevity.com/blog/is-intermittent-fasting-the-key-to-longevity/#:~:text=Yes%2C%20you%20can%20do%20 intermittent,improve%20your%20healthspan%20and%20lifespan

62. Intermittent fasting and chronic disease prevention. https://www.hopkinsmedicine.org/health/ wellness-and-prevention/intermittent-fasting-what-is-it-and-how-does-it-work#:~:text=%E2%80%9CMany%20things%20happen%20 during%20intermittent,many%20cancers%2C%E2%80%9D%20he%20 says

63. Anabolic hormonal stimulus from sets of 8–12 with 1–2 minutes of rest. https://www.ncbi.nlm.nih.gov/pmc/articles/PMC4461225/

Acknowledgments

First, I must thank my family for putting up with me. It has taken 23 years of this work to realize what it truly means to help others and prioritize what is important to me. You have always been there for me and waited for me to figure out the right balance. Thank you! I love you all so much! My kids are Ari, Asher, Aven, and Arke. You inspire me, and I always want to be your role model. Christine, you are my partner in marriage and work. I couldn't ask for a better person for both. My parents have always been there for me during my ups and downs, and I want to thank them for their fantastic support. My sister, Lisa, and brother, Randy, have always put up with me, and no matter how badly I mess up, I always feel your love and caring support.

Not a day goes by that I don't talk to my best friend, Ethan Zohn, who has trusted me with his health and fitness over the past 15 years, even as he battled cancer twice and made comebacks to compete in CBS's *Survivor*, run marathons, and play soccer again. Your friendship means the world to me.

A huge thanks to my community at Fit Studio in Minneapolis. You have been there since the beginning and have given me the opportunity to create a Blue Zone of fitness in our little community. Your support through everything and belief in me and Christine and our vision is a big part of what has kept me going.

Juliette Starrett, thank you for the work you and Kelly do. We can all learn from you. You have gone out of your way to take my calls and text messages when I needed help and support.

Stacy Anderson, thank you for taking a chance on me at Anytime Fitness Corporate HQ, showing me a larger world of fitness, and being open to my crazy ideas and views. Your support gave me the confidence to write this book.

Buzz Lagos was my coach for eight years while I was a professional soccer player. You were ahead of your time. You were a role model for how to coach, be prepared for each training session, and deal with athletes professionally and emotionally.

When I started writing this book, I wasn't sure exactly what the process would be like. I quickly learned that it was a massive undertaking, and I could not have done this without Kate Hopper, who put countless hours in at all times of the day and night to help guide, redirect, and show me the ropes of authorship.

Thank you to Delia Berrigan, my agent, who initially took a chance on me. You are always there to answer my questions, point me in the right direction, and walk me through the process.

Bill Ames, Noah Amstadter, Jesse Jordan, and the rest of the crew at Triumph Books, thank you for helping me and supporting me to get this book out in the world. It was a pleasure working with you, and I appreciate your time, effort, and knowledge.

There are so many others who helped me not only complete this book, but supported the concepts on which it is based, and without you, none of this would be possible. Thank you.